ONCOLOGY

International Journal of Cancer Research and Treatment

Founded 1948 as 'Oncologia' by H.R. Schinz
Continued by V. Richards 1967–1975

KARGER

Printed in Switzerland
on acid-free paper by
Reinhardt Druck, Basel

Appears bimonthly:
1 volume per year (6 issues)

ONCOLOGY

Submission: Only original papers written in English are considered and should be sent to:

S. Karger AG
Editorial Dept. 'Oncology'
P.O. Box
CH-4009 Basel (Switzerland)

Manuscripts should be submitted in triplicate (with three sets of illustrations of which one is an original), typewritten double-spaced on one side of the paper, with a wide margin.

Conditions: All manuscripts are subject to editorial review. The editors reserve the right to improve style and, if necessary, return the manuscript for re-writing to the author. Submission of an article for publication implies the transfer of the copyright from the author to the publisher upon acceptance. Accepted papers become the permanent property of 'Oncology' and may not be reproduced by any means, in whole or in part, without the written consent of the publisher. It is the author's responsibility to obtain permission to reproduce illustrations, tables, etc. from other publications.

Arrangement

Title page: The first page of each paper should indicate the title (main title underlined), the authors' names, and the institute where the work was conducted. A short title for use as running head as well as the full address of the author to whom correspondence should be sent are also required.
Full address: The exact postal address complete with postal code must be given at the bottom of the title page. Please also supply Phone and Fax numbers.
Key words: For indexing purposes, a list of 3-10 key words in English is essential.
Abstract: Each paper needs an abstract of up to 10 lines.
Small type: Paragraphs which can or must be set in smaller type (case histories, test methods, etc.) should be indicated with a 'p' (petit) in the margin on the left-hand side.
Footnotes: Avoid footnotes. When essential, they are numbered consecutively and typed at the foot of the appropriate page.
Tables and illustrations: Tables and illustrations (both numbered in Arabic numerals) should be prepared on separate sheets. Tables require a heading and figures a legend, also prepared on a separate sheet. For the reproduction of illustrations, only good drawings and original photographs can be accepted; negatives or photocopies cannot be used. When possible, group several illustrations on one block for reproduction (max. size 181 × 223 mm) or provide crop marks. On the back of each illustration, indicate its number, the author's name, and 'top'. Color illustrations are reproduced at the author's expense.
References: In the text identify references by Arabic numerals [in square brackets]. Material submitted for publication but not yet accepted should be noted as 'unpublished data' and not be included in the reference list. The list of references should include only those publications which are cited in the text. Do not alphabetize; number references in the order in which they are first mentioned in the text. The surnames of the authors followed by initials should be given. There should be no punctuation other than a comma to separate the authors. Cite all authors, 'et al' is not sufficient. Abbreviate journal names according to the Index Medicus system. (Also see International Committee of Medical Journal Editors: Uniform requirements for manuscripts submitted to biomedical journals. Br Med J 1988;296:401-405.)
Examples
(a) Papers published in periodicals: Kauffman HF, van der Heide S, Beaumont F, Blok H, de Vries K: Class-specific antibody determination against *Aspergillus fumigatus* by means of the enzyme-linked immunosorbent assay. III. Comparative study: IgG, IgA, IgM ELISA titers, precipitating antibodies and IgE binding after fractionation of the antigen. Int Arch Allergy Appl Immunol 1986;80:300-306.
(b) Monographs: Matthews DE, Farewell VT: Using and Understanding Medical Statistics. Basel, Karger, 1985.
(c) Edited books: Hardy WD Jr, Essex M: FeLV-induced feline acquired immune deficiency syndrome: A model for human AIDS; in Klein E (ed): Acquired Immunodeficiency Syndrome. Prog Allergy. Basel, Karger, 1986, vol 37, pp 353-376.
Further details: Authors may consult our leaflet 'Rules for the Preparation of Manuscripts', available on request from the Publisher, S. Karger AG, P.O. Box, CH-4009 Basel (Switzerland).

Page charges: There is no page charge for papers of 3 or fewer printed pages (including tables, illustrations and references). Each additional complete or partial page is charged to the author at SFr. 225.– / US$ 150.00. The allotted size of a paper is equal to approx. 9 manuscript pages (including tables, illustrations and references).

Galley proofs: Unless indicated otherwise, galley proofs are sent to the first-named author and should be returned with the least possible delay. Alterations made in galley proofs, other than the correction of printer's errors, are charged to the author. No page proofs are supplied.

Reprints: Order forms and a price list are sent with the galley proofs. Orders submitted after the issue is printed are subject to considerably higher prices. Allow five weeks from date of publication for delivery of reprints.

KARGER

General Information

ONCOLOGY

Publication data: 'Oncology' is published 6 times annually. Volume 50 with 6 issues appears in 1993.

Subscription rates: Subscriptions run for a full calendar year. Prices are given per volume.

Personal subscription:

Subscription + postage and handling

SFr. 555.10 + SFr. 16.80 Europe

SFr. 555.10 + SFr. 25.20 Overseas

US$ 370.30 + US$ 16.80

(Must be in the name of, billed to, and paid by an individual. Order must be marked 'personal subscription'.)

Institutional subscription:

Subscription + postage and handling

SFr. 793.– + SFr. 24.– Europe

SFr. 793.– + SFr. 36.– Overseas

US$ 529.00 + US$ 24.00

Airmail postage: SFr. 36.–, US$ 30.00. (Extra per volume.)

Microform edition: SFr. 396.50, US$ 264.50. (Available exclusively to subscribers of the paper edition.)

Advertising: Correspondence and rate requests should be addressed to the Publisher.

Subscription orders: Orders can be placed at agencies, bookstores, directly with the Publisher S. Karger AG, P.O. Box, CH–4009 Basel (Switzerland) or with any of the following distributors:

Deutschland: S. Karger GmbH
Lörracher Strasse 16A, Postfach
D-W-7800 Freiburg

France: Librairie Luginbühl
36, bd de Latour-Maubourg, F-75007 Paris

Great Britain, Ireland: S. Karger Publishers
11 Ravenscroft Road
Beckenham, Kent BR3 4TP

USA: S. Karger Publishers, Inc.
26 West Avon Road, P.O. Box 529
Farmington, CT 06085

India, Bangladesh, Sri Lanka:
S. Karger India Subscription Agency
B – 5/132 Safdarjung Enclave
New Delhi-110029

Japan: Katakura Libri, Inc.
36-9 Hongo 3-chome, Bunkyo-ku, Tokyo 113

Change of address: Both old and new address should be sent to the subscription source.

Single issues and back volumes: Information can be obtained through the Publisher.

Bibliographic indices: This journal is regularly listed in bibliographic services, including *Current Contents®*.

Book Reviews: Books are accepted for review by special agreement.

KARGER

Contributions to Oncology/Beiträge zur Onkologie
(ISSN 0250–3220), **Vol. 43**
Series Editors: H. Huber, Innsbruck; W. Queisser, Mannheim

H.-H. Sedlacek, G. Seemann, D. Hoffmann,
J. Czech, P. Lorenz, C. Kolar, K. Bosslet

Antibodies as Carriers of Cytotoxicity

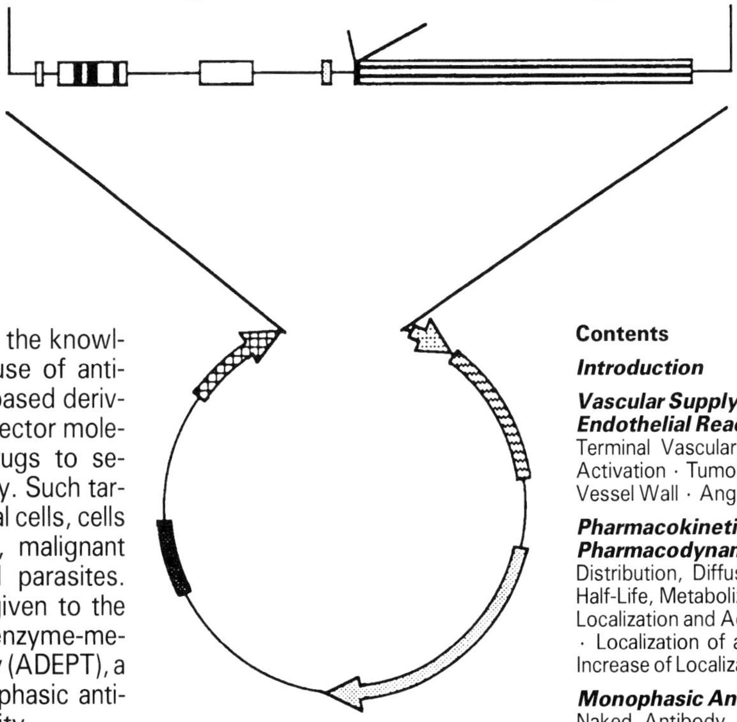

This review describes the knowledge to date in the use of antibodies and antibody-based derivatives for targeting effector molecules of cytotoxic drugs to selected cells in the body. Such target cells may be normal cells, cells infected with viruses, malignant cells or bacteria and parasites. Special emphasis is given to the antibody-dependent enzyme-mediated prodrug therapy (ADEPT), a recently developed biphasic antibody treatment modality.
By critically reviewing the perspectives of monoclonal antibodies in therapy, this volume provides stimulating reading for oncologists, pharmacologists and researchers in internal medicine.

Fields of Interest

Oncology; Immunology; Angiology, Chemotherapy, Enzymology, Pharmacokinetics, Pharmacology, Radiology, Toxicology

Contents

Contributions to Oncology/Beiträge zur Onkologie, Vol. 43
Sedlacek, H.-H. (Marburg) et al.
Antibodies as Carriers of Cytotoxicity
VIII + 208 p., 19 fig., 47 tab., hard cover, 1992
SFr. 82.– / DM 98.– / £ 41.00 / US$ 65.75
Prices subject to change
DM price for FRG, £ price for UK, US $ price for USA only
ISBN 3–8055–5599–7

KI 92613

KARGER

Recent Advances in the Usage of Mitomycin

Proceedings of a Symposium
Held in Hawaii
March 21–24, 1991

Guest Editor:
I. Craig Henderson
San Francisco, Calif.

5 figures and 56 tables, 1993

KARGER

Oncology

Vol. 50, Supplement 1, 1993

Supported by an unrestricted educational grant from
Bristol-Myers Squibb Company and Kyowa Hakko

S. Karger
Medical and Scientific Publishers
Basel · Freiburg · Paris · London
New York · New Delhi · Bangkok
Singapore · Tokyo · Sydney

Drug Dosage
The authors and the publisher have exerted every effort to ensure that drug selection and dosage set forth in this text are in accord with current recommendations and practice at the time of publication. However, in view of ongoing research, changes in government regulations, and the constant flow of information relating to drug therapy and drug reactions, the reader is urged to check the package insert for each drug for any change in indications and dosage and for added warnings and precautions. This is particularly important when the recommended agent is a new and/or infrequently employed drug.

Printed in Switzerland on acid-free paper by
Reinhardt Druck, Basel
ISBN 3-8055-5775-2

Contents

Oncology 1993;50(suppl 1):1–8

Gabriel N. Hortobagyi

Department of Medical Oncology,
Breast Medical Oncology Service,
The University of Texas M. D. Anderson
Cancer Center, Houston, Tex., USA

Mitomycin: Its Evolving Role in the Treatment of Breast Cancer

Key Words
Mitomycin
Breast cancer
Chemotherapy

Abstract
Investigators have compiled extensive experience with mitomycin in the treatment of patients with breast cancer. Given as a single agent in intermittent schedules, mitomycin has induced responses of 26–38% in previously untreated patients and of 15–25% in those exposed to multiple prior chemotherapy regimens. Duration of response has been short. Toxicity, primarily myelosuppression, is largely dose-dependent. The dose-dependent efficacy of mitomycin has not yet been addressed. Preclinical studies suggest that optimal single-agent results are obtained when mitomycin is given in intermittent, high-dose schedules. Combination chemotherapy with mitomycin has proven more effective than single-agent therapy. Mitomycin given in combination with doxorubicin produces higher response rates than have been obtained with mitomycin alone. The 3M combination (mitomycin/mitoxantrone/methotrexate) appears effective and well tolerated at the doses described. Future research should focus on the development of polychemotherapeutic regimens that can be delivered in sequential or alternating schedules. Such regimens may yield quicker responses, and thus improve survival, in patients with breast cancer.

Mitomycin, an antitumor antibiotic with a broad spectrum of activity, was isolated by Hata et al [1] from *Streptomyces caespitosus* in 1956. In experimental systems the compound was found [2] to have remarkable antitumor efficacy in a great variety of hematologic malignancies and solid tumors. In fact, its spectrum of antitumor activity was one of the broadest of any substance known at that time. Initial clinical trials with mitomycin demonstrated activity in patients with chronic leukemias, malignant lymphomas, and several epithelial tumors, including carcinomas of the gastrointestinal tract, lung, and breast. The high levels of toxicity caused by the initial dose and schedule of administration, however, limited use of the drug for several years [3, 4]. Later, mitomycin was employed in an intermittent schedule and studied as a single agent and in combination regimens in most adult human malignancies. The experience with mitomycin in the treatment of breast cancer is extensive. I will review this experience, including recent developments in advanced and metastatic breast cancer, and propose some guidelines for obtaining the maximum therapeutic benefit with this agent.

Single-Agent Trials

Early clinical investigators administered mitomycin intravenously at doses ranging from 10 to 250 μg/kg/day [3]; total doses ranged from 0.3 to 2 mg/kg. The dose-limiting toxicity was thrombocytopenia or leukopenia, or both.

Gabriel N. Hortobagyi, MD
The University of Texas M.D. Anderson Cancer Center
Department of Medical Oncology
Breast Medical Oncology Service
1515 Holcombe Boulevard, Houston, TX 77030 (USA)

0030–2414/93/0507–0001
$2.75/0

Table 1. Activity of single-agent mitomycin administered in intermittent schedules

Author	Ref.	Dose/Schedule	Patients n	Responders n	Responders %
Wise et al.	6	20–30 mg,	54	14	26
		then 10–20 mg q4–6wk	18	8	44
De Lena et al.	9	20 mg/m^2 q6wk	22	5	23
Creech et al.	10	10 mg/m^2 q4wk	90	16	18
Lopez et al.	11	20 mg/m^2 q6wk	43	0	0
Pasterz et al.	12	20 mg/m^2 q6wk	43	8	19
Amiel et al.	13	20 mg/m^2 q6wk	11	2	18
Morgan	14	10 mg/m^2 q6wk	46	8	18
Walters et al.	15	20 mg/m^2, then 5–20 mg/m^2 q6wk	67	13	19

q = Every; wk = weeks.

Toxicity was dose-dependent, although individual variations in the daily dose produced myelosuppression 2 weeks after the initiation of therapy and exacerbated thrombocytopenia to a severe degree after 3$^1/_2$ weeks. Recovery took 2–3 weeks longer requiring a corresponding delay of therapy. The very first clinical trial [3] with mitomycin showed a demonstrable antitumor effect in 4 of 7 patients with metastatic breast cancer. In 2 of these patients the effect persisted for several months. Because of severe toxicity, including toxic deaths, related to the initially employed daily schedule of administration, other dose schedules were explored. Reviewing the early Japanese studies of single-agent mitomycin activity, Frank and Osterberg [4] noted that 26 patients with breast cancer were treated at doses of 1–7 mg/day for 4–85 days. Eleven of the 26 (42%) had some objective evidence of response. A weekly schedule of administration was initiated by Hum et al [5], who reported their experience with 54 evaluable patients. Because of progressive toxicity, the starting dose (10 mg/m^2/week) was decreased to 5 mg/m^2/week. Despite this reduction, hematologic toxicity remained dose-limiting, and the weekly schedule yielded no advantages over the previously described daily schedule. Although response rates as high as 67% have been reported [6], large reviews [2, 7, 8] of pooled data from multiple studies have placed the response rate to intermittently administered single-agent mitomycin in patients with metastatic breast cancer at between 26 and 38% (table 1) [6, 9–15]. Not surprisingly, for patients exposed to multiple prior chemotherapy regimens, the response rate has been lower, ranging from 15 to 25% [11, 12, 15].

Dose- and Schedule-Related Issues

Experimental studies suggested a steep dose-response relationship for mitomycin in preclinical systems [16]. The dose-dependent efficacy of mitomycin in humans has not yet been addressed. Retrospective analyses of open phase II trials suggest that doses of 10–20 mg/m^2 given every 4–6 weeks yield similar results. In fact, the only randomized comparison of single-agent mitomycin with doxorubicin used the former at a dose of 10 mg/m^2 given every 6 weeks, half the maximally tolerated dose (MTD) for this schedule [14]. The doxorubicin dose was 50 mg/m^2 given every 3 weeks, which also was lower than the MTD for this schedule. At these doses and schedules the 2 drugs were equivalent, producing objective regressions in 18% of patients. Most responses occurred during the first treatment cycle.

Myelosuppressive toxicity is cumulative and related to cumulative dose. Thus, it was hypothesized that low doses of mitomycin producing antitumor efficacy similar to that obtained with higher doses would be better tolerated and could stretch the drug's useful life. With this in mind, Walters et al. [15] undertook a randomized trial in which patients with metastatic breast cancer were treated initially with mitomycin 20 mg/m^2 i.v. and subsequently randomly assigned to maintenance therapy with either 20 mg/m^2 i.v. every 6 weeks or 5 mg/m^2 i.v. every 6 weeks. After 67 evaluable patients completed the trial, the two treatment arms showed no detectable difference in response rate or remission duration. Severe toxicity, however, was limited to the high-dose maintenance arm. Thus, it is likely that doses of mitomycin lower than those ordinarily used could be used successfully, especially in combination chemotherapy.

Higher-than-standard doses of mitomycin (up to 120 mg/m^2) have also been explored [17–19] in phase I dose-escalation studies with and without autologous bone marrow support. The number of patients with breast carcinoma included in these studies has been relatively small (table 2), and results do not show a marked increase in efficacy for mitomycin doses higher than 20 mg/m^2. Toxicity, however, was considerably increased and included pulmonary, renal, gut, and hepatic toxicities, as well as several toxic deaths. Most investigators [18, 19] concluded that extramedullary toxicities preclude the use of mitomycin in high doses.

Because of mitomycin's relatively short half-life in plasma, clinical studies have evaluated administration of mitomycin by 24-hour continuous intravenous infusion [20], by 120-hour continuous intravenous infusion [21], and via infusions lasting 9–30 days [22]. Regardless of the duration of infusion, the dose-limiting toxicity in all cases was myelosuppression, whereas nausea, vomiting, and renal toxicities were markedly decreased. The number of patients entered into these trials was too small to assess therapeutic efficacy compared with standard intermittent, high-dose administration. Preclinical studies, however, suggested that mitomycin given in intermittent, high-dose schedules produces optimal results [23].

Combination Studies

Evaluation of pooled data [24] of single-agent therapy in patients with breast cancer revealed that mitomycin and doxorubicin are the two most effective single agents. Combination therapy, however, is clearly more effective than single-agent chemotherapy in such patients. Although single-agent mitomycin produces responses in a substantial fraction of patients, the duration of these responses is short. Consequently, several combinations containing mitomycin and doxorubicin were developed and studied, with the aim of increasing efficacy with tolerable toxicity. Table 3 shows results obtained with combinations containing both agents [13, 14, 25–35]. In some reports the combination was restricted to patients without prior chemotherapy, whereas in others the combination was administered to patients who had relapsed from front-line treatment with other standard agents. Most cytotoxic agents, mitomycin and doxorubicin included, are more effective in patients without prior chemotherapy exposure. Not surprisingly, then, mitomycin/doxorubicin-containing combinations were found to be more effective in previously untreated patients [13, 14, 26, 33] than in second-line or salvage situations. [13, 27–29, 33]. Even in previously treated patients, however, these combinations have been as effective as any other standard-dose combination or second- or third-line therapies available today. Mitomycin/doxorubicin-containing combinations induce longer durations of response than does single-agent mitomycin, and offer substantial palliation to many patients.

Other frequently used regimens combine mitomycin with one of the vinca alkaloids, mostly vinblastine or vindesine. Table 4 summarizes published information about these combinations [36–49]. Although additional drugs were included in some combinations, mitomycin and vinca alkaloid comprised the basic nucleus. Vincristine in combination with mitomycin does not appear to be more effective than mitomycin alone, which confirms the relative lack of efficacy of vincristine observed in other combinations.

Mitomycin was also combined with antimetabolites like methotrexate [43, 50] or 5-fluorouracil (5-FU) [47, 48]. These combinations appear active too, although there are no controlled studies to show their superiority over single-agent chemotherpy. With the exception of myelosuppression, the toxicity of the antimetabolites is quite different from that of mitomycin; therefore, the two types of agents can be combined at close to the maximally tolerated doses.

Although mitomycin/doxorubicin-containing combinations were effective, increased rates of cardiac toxicity were also observed [51]. This prompted investigators to study combinations of mitomycin with mitoxantrone, an anthraquinone with antitumor activity similar to that of doxorubicin, but with decreased cardiotoxic potential. The reported results of mitomycin/mitoxantrone combination chemotherapy are shown in table 5 [42, 45, 46, 52]. Unfortunately, the varied patient selection, drug doses, and schedules of administration used in these trials make it difficult to compare results with those obtained using

Table 2. Response to high-dose mitomycin in metastatic breast cancer

Author	Ref.	Dose/Schedule	Patients n	Responders	
				n	%
Godfrey	8	50 mg, then 10–30 mg q4–6wk	9	4	44
Tannir et al.	18	20 mg/m², then 30–50 mg/m² + ABMT	8	1	12.5
Tannir et al.	18	40 mg/m² q6wk	7	–	–
Karanes et al.	19	60 mg/m²	2	1	50

ABMT = Autologous bone marrow transplantation; q = every; wk = weeks.

Table 3. Combination chemotherapy with mitomycin and doxorubicin for metastatic breast cancer

Author	Ref.	Agent	Dose mg/m²	Schedule	Patients n	Response %	Response duration months
Creech et al.	25	Mitomycin Doxorubicin	10 i.v. d1 20 i.v. d1,8	q28d	71	51	7
Amiel et al.	13	Mitomycin Doxorubicin	10 i.v. d1 40 i.v. d1	q21d	27	59	9
Morgan	14	Mitomycin Doxorubicin	5–10 i.v. d1 30–50 i.v. d1,21	q42d	27	41	6+
Harris et al.	26	Mitomycin Doxorubicin	10 i.v. d1 40 i.v. d1,21	q42d	24	25	9.6
Varini et al.	27	Mitomycin Doxorubicin Vincristine	10 i.v. d1 45 i.v. d1,29 1.2 i.v. d1,29	q56d	47	34	NA
Shipp et al.	28	Mitomycin Doxorubicin Vincristine	10 i.v. d1 40 i.v. d1,21 1.5 i.v. d1,21	q42d	36	31	5
Luikart et al.	29	Mitomycin Doxorubicin Vinblastine	10 i.v. d1 30 i.v. d1,28 6 i.v. d1,28	q56d	27	33	4
Pinnamaneni et al.	30	Mitomycin Doxorubicin Dibromodulcitol	10 i.v. d1 40 i.v. d1 70 p.o. d1–6, 23–27	q42d	26	54	10
Borovik et al.	31	Mitomycin Doxorubicin Vinblastine	10 i.v. d1 45 i.v. d1,21 4.5 i.v. d1,21	q42d	31	24	6
Sulkes et al.	32	Mitomycin Doxorubicin Vinblastine	10 i.v. d1 20 i.v. d1,8,15 6 i.v. d1,8,15	q42d	36	28	10
Oster et al.	33	Mitomycin Doxorubicin Vincristine	10 i.v. d1 50 i.v. d1,28 1 i.v. d1,28	q56d	15	73	8
Friedman et al.	34	Mitomycin Doxorubicin Vincristine 5-FU	10 i.v. d1 40 i.v. d1,28 1 i.v. d1,28 400 i.v. d1,8,28,36	q56d	82	35	7
Anderson et al.	35	Mitomycin Doxorubicin	10 i.v. d1 45 i.v. d1,21	q42d	39	49	10

NA = Not available; d = days.

Table 4. Combination chemotherapy including mitomycin and agents other than doxorubicin

Author	Ref.	Agent	Dose mg/m^2	Schedule	Patients n	Response %	Response duration months
Radford et al.	36	Mitomycin	12 i.v. d1	q21d	40	28	5
		Vinblastine	6 i.v. d1				
Garewel et al.	37	Mitomycin	10 i.v. d1,28	q42–56d	22	32	5
		Vinblastine	5 i.v. d1,14,28,42				
Konits et al.	38	Mitomycin	20 i.v. d1	q42–56d	30	40	4
		Vinblastine	0.15[1] i.v. d1,21				
Brambilla et al.	39	Mitomycin	10 i.v. d1	q28d	44	23	7
		Vinblastine	5 i.v. d1,15				
Howell et al.	40	Mitomycin	10 i.v. d1	q28d	24	66	NA
		Vinblastine	10 i.v. d1				
		Dibromodulcitol	500 p.o. daily				
Chauvergne et al.	41	Mitomycin	10 i.v. d1	q21d	100	15	8
		Vindesine	4 i.v. d1				
		Thiotepa	20 i.v. d1				
Belpomme et al.	42	Mitomycin	8 i.v. d1	q56d	46	34	14+
		Vindesine	2.5 i.v. d1,8,29,36				
		Mitoxantrone	12 i.v. d1,29				
Pouillart et al.	43	Mitomycin	10 i.v. d2	q21d	56	30	8
		Methotrexate	12.5 i.v. d2,3	(q12h)			
		Teniposide	100 i.v. d22				
Garewel et al.	37	Mitomycin	10 i.v. d1,28	q42–56d	15	40	8
		Vindesine	2 i.v. d1,14,28,42				
Costanzo et al.	44	Mitomycin	12 i.v. d1	q42d	31	16	15
		Vindesine	3 i.v. d1,8,15,22,28,35				
Perren et al.	45	Mitomycin	6 i.v. d1	q21d	13	46	8+
		Mitoxantrone	12 i.v. d1				
		Vincristine	2 i.v. d1				
Bishop et al.	46	Mitomycin	10–15 i.v. d1	q42d	56	18	7+
		Mitoxantrone	8–10 i.v. d1,21				
Mattson et al.	47	Mitomycin	6 i.v. d2	q21d	50	58	NA
		5-FU	1,000 i.v. d132				
Aspegren and Landbert	48	Mitomycin	6 i.v. d1	q21d	53	16.5	NA
		5-FU	1,000 i.v. d1,2				
Perez et al.	50	Mitomycin	10 i.v. d1	q42d	48	40	5
		Melphalan	6 p.o. d1–3,22–24				
		Methotrexate	35 i.v. d1–22				

NA = Not available; d = days.
[1] mg/kg.

mitomycin/doxorubicin combinations. Cardiac toxicity, however, was only rarely observed in patients given mitomycin/mitoxantrone combinations. Controlled trials will have to be performed to determine the relative efficacy and toxicities of mitomycin combinations containing either doxorubicin or mitoxantrone.

The recently developed '3M' combination (mitomycin/mitoxantrone/methotrexate) appears to be effective against metastatic breast cancer and well tolerated at the doses described [52]. Acute toxicities are less prominent than those observed with more commonly used combinations like FAC (5-FU/doxorubicin/cyclophosphamide) and CMF (cyclophosphamide/methotrexate/5-FU). Only one comparative trial of 3M versus VAC (vincristine/doxorubicin/cyclophosphamide) has been performed and suggested therapeutic equivalence with better tolerance for the 3M combination [52].

Table 5. Mitomycin/mitoxantrone-containing combinations for advanced breast cancer

Author	Ref.	Agent	Dose/Schedule	Patients n	Response %
Belpomme et al.	42	Mitomycin Mitoxantrone Vindesine	8 mg/m^2 i.v. q8wk 12 mg/m^2 i.v. q4wk 2.5 mg/m^2 i.v. days 1,8,29,36	46	34
Perren et al.	45	Mitomycin Mitoxantrone Vincristine	6 mg/m^2 i.v. q3wk 12 mg/m^2 i.v. q3wk 2 mg i.v. q3wk	13	46
Bishop et al.	46	Mitomycin Mitoxantrone	10–15 mg/m^2 i.v. q6wk 8–10 mg/m^2 i.v. q3wk	56	18
Judson et al.	52	Mitomycin Mitoxantrone Methotrexate	7 mg/m^2 i.v. q6wk 7 mg/m^2 i.v. q3wk 30 mg/m^2 i.v. q3wk	61	56

wk = Weeks.

Combinations of mitomycin with other cytotoxic agents have been used less frequently. The combinations described above are by and large the most useful to date, and certainly their therapeutic ratios have been well established.

Toxicity

Administered at 15–20 mg/m^2 i.v. every 6 weeks, mitomycin is very well tolerated and has few acute side effects. The dose-limiting toxicity of mitomycin and mitomycin-containing combinations is cumulative myelosuppression, especially thrombocytopenia. Although initial myelosuppression is moderate, cumulative thrombocytopenia appears after the second or third dose. This effect is related to cumulative dose and not to schedule of administration.

Mitomycin's acute side effects are less frequent and severe than those of many other cytotoxic agents used against breast cancer. Nausea and vomiting, while possible, occur infrequently and are rarely severe. Mucositis and diarrhea are minor side effects observed in less than 20% of patients. Anorexia is common, and its severity increases with cumulative doses. Severe toxicity is fortunately observed in a small minority of patients. Upon extravasation mitomycin can cause severe skin ulceration similar to that observed with doxorubicin [53]. Interstitial pneumonitis and pulmonary fibrosis, as well as renal failure and microangiopathic hemolytic uremic syndrome, have been observed [7]. Pulmonary and renal complications appear related to cumulative dose. Retrospective reviews have placed the critical dose above that at which toxicity occurs, i.e., at 30–60 mg/m^2 for renal toxicity [54, 55] and 20 mg/m^2 or more for mitomycin-induced pneumonitis [56]. Even at these higher cumulative doses, however, the incidence of these complications is less than 10%.

Discussion

Mitomycin, administered as a single agent and in combination chemotherapy, has clear antitumor efficacy against metastatic breast cancer. Mitomycin should not be used chronically, since dose-limiting toxicity, cumulative myelosuppression, and major organ toxicities (renal and pulmonary) appear related to cumulative dose. On the other hand, because mitomycin is one of the two most effective agents currently available for breast cancer, the toxic effects described should not preclude its use in induction regimens. As such, mitomycin-containing combinations should be compared or combined with other leading combinations in metastatic breast cancer. Over the last 15 years it has become apparent that the greatest benefit from combination chemotherapy is derived during the first 6 months of treatment. Lengthy treatment programs with the same drugs are unlikely to result in substantial improvement compared to short, intensive programs. The Goldie-Coldman [57] hypothesis suggests that early introduction of multiple effective agents will delay the appearance of clinical resistance. Therefore, it is desirable to develop several effective polychemotherapy regimens against metastatic (or even early) breast cancer. These regimens should lack cross-resistance, and the use of one should not preclude the use of others. The sequential or alternating use of these various drug regimens may lead to improved response rates and survival duration. Their most important application might be in the treatment of primary breast cancer. In fact, the 3M regimen has been reported to have a much greater degree of efficacy (response rate >80%) when used as neoadjuvant chemotherapy than against metastatic breast cancer [49]. Additional evaluation of this and other mitomycin-containing regimens is warranted.

Acknowledgment

The author thanks Rose Mary Fonseca for her assistance in the preparation of this manuscript.

References

1 Hata T, Sano Y, Sugawara R, et al: Mitomycin, a new antibiotic from streptomyces. Int J Antibiot (A) 1956;4:141–146.

2 Crooke ST, Bradner WT: Mitomycin C: A review. Cancer Treat Rev 1976;3:121–139.

3 Jones R: Mitomycin C – a preliminary report of studies of human pharmacology and initial therapeutic trial. Cancer Chemother Rep 1959;2:3–7.

4 Frank W, Osterberg AE: Mitomycin C (NSC-26980) – an evaluation of the Japanese reports. Cancer Chemother Rep 1960;9:114–119.

5 Hum GJ, Bogdon DL, Bateman JR: Phase I–II evaluation of weekly mitomycin-C (NSC-26980) for patients with metastatic GI and breast malignancies. Oncology 1974;30: 236–243.

6 Wise GR, Kuhn IN, Godfrey TE: Mitomycin C in large infrequent doses in breast cancer. Med Pediatr Oncol 1976;2:55–60.

7 Doll DC, Weiss RB, Issell BF: Mitomycin: Ten years after approval for marketing. J Clin Oncol 1985;3:276–286.

8 Godfrey TE: Mitomycin C in advanced breast cancer: An update. Semin Oncol 1988;15: 71–73.

9 De Lena M, Brillo A, Brambilla C, et al: Mitomycin C in metastatic breast cancer resistant to hormone therapy and conventional chemotherapy. Tumori 1980;66:481–487.

10 Creech RH, Catalano RB, Shah MK, et al: An effective low-dose mitomycin regimen for hormonal- and chemotherapy-refractory patients with metastatic breast cancer. Cancer 1983;51: 1034–1040.

11 Lopez M, Papaldo P, Di Lauro L, et al: Mitomycin C in patients with metastatic breast cancer refractory to hormone therapy and chemotherapy. Oncology 1983;40:244–247.

12 Pasterz RB, Buzdar AU, Hortobagyi GN, et al: Mitomycin in metastatic breast cancer refractory to hormonal and combination chemotherapy. Cancer 1985;56:2381–2384.

13 Amiel SA, Stewart JF, Earl HM, et al: Adriamycin and mitomycin C as initial chemotherapy for advanced breast cancer. Eur J Cancer Clin Oncol 1985;20(5):631–634.

14 Morgan LR: Adriamycin and mitomycin C in advanced breast cancer, in Carter SK, Crooke ST (eds): Mitomycin C: Current Status and New Developments. New York, Academic Press, 1979, pp 101–111.

15 Walters R, Frye D, Hortobagyi G: Phase II study of two dosages of mitomycin C in metastatic breast cancer (abstract). Proc Am Assoc Cancer Res 1990;31:181.

16 Dorr RT, Bowden GT, Alberts DS, et al: Interactions of mitomycin C with mammalian DNA detected by alkaline elution. Cancer Res 1985;45:3510–3516.

17 Lazarus HM, Gottfried MR, Herzig RH, et al: Veno-occlusive disease of the liver after high-dose mitomycin C therapy and autologous bone marrow transplantation. Cancer 1982; 49:1789–1795.

18 Tannir N, Spitzer G, Dicke K, et al: Phase I–II study of high-dose mitomycin with autologous bone marrow transplantation in refractory metastatic breast cancer. Cancer Treat Rep 1984;68:805–806.

19 Karanes C, Ratanatharathorn V, Schilcher RB, et al: High-dose mitomycin C with autologous bone marrow transplantation in patients with refractory malignancies. Am J Clin Oncol 1986;9:444–448.

20 Miller E, Sullivan RD, Chryssochoos T: The clinical effects of mitomycin C by continuous intravenous administration. Cancer Chemother Rep 1962;21:129–135.

21 Yap HY, Valdivieso M, Blumenschein G, et al: A phase I–II study of continuous 5-day infusion mitomycin-C. Am J Clin Oncol Cancer Clin Trials 1983;6:109–112.

22 Lokich J, Perri J, Fine N, et al: Mitomycin C: Phase I study of a constant infusion ambulatory treatment schedule. Am J Clin Oncol Cancer Clin Trials 1982;5:443–447.

23 Rockwell S, Nierenburg M, Irvin CG: Effects of the mode of administration of mitomycin on tumor and marrow response and on the therapeutic ratio. Cancer Treat Rep 1987;71:927–934.

24 Carter SK: Single and combination nonhormonal chemotherapy in breast cancer. Cancer 1972;30:1543–1555.

25 Creech RH, Dayal H, Catalano RB, et al: Combination doxorubicin-mitomycin therapy for hormonal and CMF-refractory metastatic breast cancer (abstract). Proc Am Soc Clin Oncol 1984;3:126.

26 Harris MA, Byrne PJ, Smith F, et al: Treatment of advanced breast cancer with two doxorubicin-containing regimens. Am J Clin Oncol 1984;7:51–58.

27 Varini M, Brunner K, Mermillod M, et al: DAV (dibromodulcitol, Adriamycin, vincristine) vs MAV (mitomycin-C, Adriamycin, vincristine) in advanced breast cancer (BC) (abstract No. 271). Cancer Immunol Immunother 1984;18:S68.

28 Shipp SK, Muss HB, Westrick MA, et al: Vincristine, doxorubicin and mitomycin (VAM) in patients with advanced breast cancer previously treated with cyclophosphamide, methotrexate and fluorouracil (CMF): A clinical trial of Piedmont Oncology Association (POA). Cancer Chemother Pharmacol 1983;11:130–133.

29 Luikart SD, Witman GB, Portlock CS: Adriamycin (doxorubicin), vinblastine, and mitomycin-C combination chemotherapy in refractory breast cancer. Cancer 1984;54:1252–1255.

30 Pinnamaneni K, Yap HY, Buzdar AU, et al: Adriamycin, dibromodulcitol, and mitomycin combination chemotherapy for patients with metastatic breast carcinoma previously treated with cyclophosphamide, methotrexate, 5-fluorouracil, vincristine, and prednisone. Cancer 1984;53:1841–1844.

31 Borovik R, Epelbaum R, Cohen Y, et al: Mitomycin, doxorubicin and vinblastine as second-line chemotherapy in patients with advanced breast cancer. Cancer Treat Rep 1986; 70:517–518.

32 Sulkes A, Gez E, Pfeffer R, et al: Adriamycin, vinblastine and mitomycin-C as second-line chemotherapy in advanced breast cancer. Cancer Chemother Pharmacol 1986;18:162–167.
33 Oster MW, Park Y: Vincristine, Adriamycin, and mitomycin (VAM) therapy for previously treated breast cancer. Cancer 1983;51:203–205.
34 Friedman MA, Marcus FS, Cassidy MJ: 5-fluorouracil + Oncovin + Adriamycin + mitomycin-C (FOAM): An effective program for breast cancer, even for disease refractory to previous chemotherapy. Cancer 1983;52:193–197.
35 Anderson M, Daugaard S, von der Maase H, et al: Doxorubicin versus mitomycin versus doxorubicin plus mitomycin in advanced breast cancer: A randomized study. Cancer Treat Rep 1986;70:1181–1185.
36 Radford JA, Knight RK, Rubens RD: Mitomycin-C and vinblastine in the treatment of advanced breast cancer. Eur J Cancer Clin Oncol 1985;21:1475–1477.
37 Garewel HS, Brooks RJ, Jones SE, et al: Treatment of advanced breast cancer with mitomycin-C combined with vinblastine or vindesine. J Clin Oncol 1983;1:772–775.
38 Konits PH, Aisner J, Van Echo DA, et al: Mitomycin-C and vinblastine chemotherapy for advanced breast cancer. Cancer 1984;48:1295–1298.
39 Brambilla C, Zambetti M, Ferrari L, et al: Mitomycin-C and vinblastine in advanced refractory breast cancer. Tumori 1989;75:141–144.
40 Howell A, Morrison JM, Bramwell VH, et al: Dibromodulcitol, mitomycin-C and vinblastine (DMV) chemotherapy in advanced breast cancer. Eur J Cancer Clin Oncol 1984;20:873–876.
41 Chauvergne J, Durand M, Brunet R, et al: Chemotherapy associating mitomycin-C, thiotepa and vindesine in advanced breast cancer. Bull Cancer 1981;68:442–448.
42 Belpomme D, Gisselbrecht C, Marty M, et al: Long duration of response induced by vindesine (V), mitoxantrone (M) and mitomycin-C (MC), (VMMC) in metastatic breast carcinoma (abstract). Proc Am Soc Clin Oncol 1987; 6:A224.
43 Pouillart P, Palangie T, Jouve M, et al: Cancers du sein métastasés. Efficacité d'une association de VM26, mitomycine C et de méthotrexate chez des malades resistants à une combinaison de 4 drogues comportant l'adriamycine. Bull Cancer (Paris) 1979;66:485–490.
44 Costanzo FD, Gori F, Tonato M, et al: Vindesine and mitomycin-C in chemotherapy refractory advanced breast cancer. Cancer 1986;57:904–907.
45 Perren TJ, Blackledge G, Mould JJ, et al: Phase II study of vincristine, mitomycin-C and mitoxantrone in advanced breast cancer: A preliminary report of response and toxicity. Invest New Drugs 1985;3:173–177.
46 Bishop JF, Raghavan D, Woods R: Mitomycin and mitoxantrone in previously treated patients with advanced breast cancer. Cancer Treat Rep 1987;71:191–193.
47 Mattson W, Von Eyben F, Hallsten L, et al: A phase II study of combined 5-fluorouracil and mitomycin C in advanced breast cancer. Cancer 1982;49:217–220.
48 Aspegren K, Landbert T: 5-Fluorouracil and mitomycin-C in advanced breast cancer. Radiother Oncol 1986;6:121–126.
49 Powles TJ, Ford HJ, Nash AG: A feasibility trial to compare chemotherapy with mitomycin C, mitoxantrone and methotrexate (3M) plus tamoxifen starting 3 months before surgery (neoadjuvant) or entirely after surgery (adjuvant) for women with primary operable breast cancer (abstract B28). 3rd Int Congr Neo-Adjuvant Chemother, Paris, 1991, p 16.
50 Perez DJ, Powles TJ, Gazet JC, et al: Mitomycin C, melphalan and methotrexate combination chemotherapy for palliation of disseminated breast cancer. Cancer Chemother Pharmacol 1984;13:36–38.
51 Villani F, Comazzi R, Lacaita G, et al: Possible enhancement of the cardiotoxicity of doxorubicin when combined with mitomycin C. Med Oncol Tumor Pharmacother 1985;2:93–97.
52 Judson IR, Powles TJ, Ashley SE, et al: Mitomycin C, mitoxantrone and methotrexate (3M) for advanced breast cancer. A randomized crossover trial versus vincristine, Adriamycin and cyclophosphamide (VAC). 3M is equally effective with reduced toxicity (abstract No. 37). Proc Am Soc Clin Oncol 1988; 7:10.
53 Argenta LC, Manders EK: Mitomycin C extravasation injuries. Cancer 1983;51:1080–1082.
54 Valavaara R, Nordman E: Renal complications of mitomycin C therapy with special reference to the total dose. Cancer 1985;55:47–50.
55 Verwey J, de Vries J, Pinedo HM: Mitomycin C-induced renal toxicity, a dose-dependent side effect? Eur J Cancer Clin Oncol 1987;23:195–199.
56 Verweij J, van Zanten T, Souren T, et al: Prospective study on the dose relationship of mitomycin C-induced interstitial pneumonitis. Cancer 1987;60:756–761.
57 Goldie JH, Coldman A: A mathematical model for relating the drug sensitivity of tumors to their spontaneous mutation rate. Cancer Treat Rep 1979;63:1727–1733.

Oncology 1993;50(suppl 1):9–15

Ian E. Smith
Trevor J. Powles

The Breast Unit, Royal Marsden Hospital, London and Surrey, UK

MMM (Mitomycin/Mitoxantrone/Methotrexate): An Effective New Regimen in the Treatment of Metastatic Breast Cancer

Key Words
Chemotherapy
Metastatic breast cancer

Abstract
MMM (mitomycin 7–8 mg/m^2 i.v.) every 6 weeks; mitoxantrone 7–8 mg/m^2 i.v. every 3 weeks; methotrexate 35 mg/m^2 i.v. every 3 weeks) is a new combination chemotherapy regimen for advanced breast cancer. It has been compared in two complementary randomized trials with CMF (cyclophosphamide 100 mg orally, days 1–14; methotrexate 35 mg/m^2 i.v. days 1 and 8; 5-fluorouracil 1 g i.v. days 1 and 8; courses repeated at 28-day intervals) and VAC (vincristine 1.4 mg/m^2 every 3 weeks, anthracycline 30 mg/m^2 every 3 weeks, cyclophosphamide 400 mg/m^2 every 3 weeks) in patients with advanced metastatic breast cancer. In the first trial, which involved 227 patients, 53% of patients receiving MMM and 49% receiving VAC responded to treatment. There was no significant difference between treatment groups in median response duration or survival. Incidence of neuropathy, alopecia, and nausea and vomiting was significantly higher in patients receiving VAC. Hematologic toxicity was greater in the MMM group. In the second trial, which involved 120 patients, 51% of patients receiving MMM and 60% receiving CMF responded to treatment. Again, there was no significant difference between treatment groups in median response duration or survival. Both regimens were well tolerated with a low incidence of alopecia and serious nausea and vomiting, and there were no significant differences in toxicity. Significant reductions in serial left ventricular ejection fractions occurred in 4 patients given CMF and in 2 given MMM. MMM is an effective, well-tolerated regimen for advanced breast cancer, with toxicity similar to that of CMF and less than that of an anthracycline-containing regimen.

In the absence of curative chemotherapy for patients with metastatic breast cancer, the search continues for new regimens that are not merely effective but have low subjective toxicity. Mitomycin is an active and well-tolerated single agent in this disease, yielding a 28% overall response rate even in previously treated patients [1]. Mitoxantrone (Novantrone), a new anthracenedione, has likewise been shown to be active and well tolerated in the treatment of metastatic breast cancer, producing overall single-agent response rates of up to 35% in previously

Ian E. Smith, MD
Royal Marsden Hospital
Downs Road
Sutton, Surrey SM2 5PT (UK)

0030–2414/93/0507–0009
$2.75/0

untreated patients [2]. A long-established and widely used drug in the treatment of breast cancer, methotrexate, has also produced a low incidence of significant toxicity. We established the regimen designated MMM (mitomycin/mitoxantrone/methotrexate) with the aim of achieving an effective palliative regimen with a low incidence of subjective toxicity and low risk of severe alopecia in patients with metastatic breast cancer. We have compared this regimen in concurrent randomized trials with the VAC (vincristine/anthracycline/cyclophosphamide) and CMF (cyclophosphamide/methotrexate/5-fluorouracil – 5-FU) regimens.

Table 1. Patient characteristics: CMF versus MMM

	CMF	MMM
Patients, n	60	60
Median age, years (range)	55 (31–72)	51 (29–80)
Menopausal status		
Pre	19	21
Peri	3	4
Post	38	35
Sites, median n (range)	2 (1–5)	2 (1–5)
Previous endocrine therapy for advanced disease	42	44
Median disease-free interval, months	24	25
Primary medical treatment	6	5
Presenting with metastatic disease	12	16

From Jodrell et al. [15], with permission.

Trial 1: MMM Versus CMF

Patient Characteristics

The Breast Unit at the Royal Marsden Hospital, London, entered into this trial 120 women with histologically or cytologically proven breast cancer and distant metastases or locally advanced inoperable disease. Details of patient characteristics are given in table 1. Median age was 55 years (range, 31–72) and 51 years (range, 29–80) for patients in the CMF and MMM groups, respectively. Among patients enrolled, 37% receiving CMF and 42% MMM were premenopausal or perimenopausal (2 years since last menstrual period). The majority of patients (70% receiving CMF and 73% MMM) had received at least one form of previous endocrine therapy for advanced disease, but no patient had received previous chemotherapy for advanced disease or as adjuvant treatment. Eleven patients (6 receiving CMF, 5 MMM) had large primary carcinomas without metastatic spread, and 28 (12 CMF, 16 MMM) had metastatic disease at initial presentation. For the remainder of patients, the median disease-free interval was 24 and 25 months for the CMF and MMM groups, respectively.

Exclusion criteria included previous cytotoxic chemotherapy; significant nonmetastatic cardiac, renal, or hepatic disease; life expectancy under 3 months; or unassessable disease as defined by standard International Union Against Cancer (UICC) criteria [3].

Randomization and Treatment Schedules

Patients were randomized to receive MMM or CMF as first-line treatment using a permutated block technique. There was no stratification. Treatment was usually given on an outpatient basis, and the chemotherapy regimens were as follows: MMM – mitoxantrone 8 mg/m^2 i.v. day 1; methotrexate 35 mg/m^2 i.v. (maximum dose, 50 mg) day 1; mitomycin 8 mg/m^2 i.v. day 1; alternate courses only were repeated every 21 days. CMF – cyclophosphamide 100 mg/m^2 orally days 1–14; methotrexate 35 mg/m^2 i.v. (maximum dose, 50 mg) days 1 and 8; 5-FU 1 g i.v. days 1 and 8; courses were repeated every 28 days. Initially, prophylactic leucovorin rescue was not used, and a significant number of patients complained of low-grade (World Health Organization – WHO – grade I or II) but troublesome mucositis. Therefore, after February 1987, leucovorin (15 mg orally every 6 h × 4, commencing 24 h after chemotherapy) was prescribed prophylactically for the 81 patients subsequently enrolled.

Treatment Duration and Crossover

Patients who achieved an objective response as defined by standard UICC criteria [3] continued receiving treatment for 6 courses and were then randomized to either stop or continue treatment for an additional 6 courses as part of a separate maintenance chemotherapy trial. If clinically appropriate, patients who developed progressive disease or had stable disease but failed to achieve symptomatic relief after 2 courses were changed to a crossover regimen excluding methotrexate (i.e., MM or CF). Likewise, responding patients received the crossover regimen at relapse.

Dose Modification

Treatment was only given if the peripheral WBC count was over 3.0×10^9/l and platelet count over 100×10^9/l. If either count was under these respective values at the start of the second or subsequent courses, treatment was delayed until these parameters recovered. After two delays the dose of each drug was reduced by 25% and if two further delays occurred, reductions to 50% of the original dose were made. Further delays resulted in the discontinuation of treatment. If any patient developed neutropenic infection, the doses of all drugs in subsequent courses were reduced by 25%.

Antiemetics

All patients received prophylactic antiemetic cover usually comprising metoclopramide 20 mg i.v. and dexamethasone 8 mg i.v. or orally prechemotherapy. If nausea or vomiting occurred, metoclopramide 20 mg was given orally every 4–6 h after the initial intravenous injection and, if necessary, lorazepam 1 mg orally every 4–6 h was added as a third agent.

Assessment of Response and Toxicity

Full clinical history and examination, peripheral full blood count, plasma urea and electrolytes, and serum liver function tests were carried out before each treatment. Specific investigations to document and assess tumor sites, including chest X-ray, radiologic skeletal survey, and computed tomography scan, were carried out prior to treatment, after 2 courses, and at the end of treatment. Palpable lesions were assessed after each course, and regular assessment of other disease sites was carried out where clinically indicated. Response was assessed according to standard UICC criteria [3]. Life tables were drawn using the Kaplan-Meier method, and comparisons were performed using the log-rank test [4]. Groups were compared using the $\chi 2$ test and the Mann-Whitney test for trend. Toxicity for each course of treatment was assessed using standard WHO criteria [5]. Because all patients in this trial received phrophylactic antiemetics, WHO criteria for nausea and vomiting were not applicable. We therefore defined a scoring system as follows: grade 1 = mild nausea/vomiting, still able to eat; grade 2 = moderate nausea with anorexia or two to three regurgitations occurring in under 24 h; grades 3–4 = severe anorexia or prolonged vomiting lasting more than 24 h.

Cardiotoxicity

Cardiac function was monitored in all patients entered after October 1986. An electrocardiogram and assessment of left ventricular ejection fraction (LVEF) at rest and during exercise were performed prior to treatment, at crossover (i.e., in cases of disease progression), and at completion of treatment. These assessments were continued at 6-month intervals during follow-up. LVEF was assessed by gated pool scanning following in vivo labeling of RBCs with technetium-99m, a technique commonly used in the assessment of anthracycline-induced cardiotoxicity [6]. One hundred seven patients were eligible for this part of the protocol, but only 75 underwent assessment. Fifteen patients were deemed too ill to complete the stress phase of the study, 16 patients were not asked to enter because of transport problems, and 1 patient suffered a cerebrovascular thromboembolism before an initial CT scan was performed.

Response Results

One hundred twelve patients were evaluable for response (55 receiving CMF, 57 MMM). Eight patients initially randomized were deemed inevaluable for response because of treatment toxicity (1 receiving CMF), unwillingness to continue (2 CMF, 1 MMM), or early death during first course of treatment (2 CMF, 2 MMM). Twenty-nine patients taking MMM achieved an objective response (51%; 95% confidence interval, CI 38–64%) compared with 33 receiving CMF (60%; 95% CI 47–73%). Of these responders, 2 (4%) in each group achieved a complete remission. No significant differences between the two groups were found for median response duration (7 months, both MMM and CMF), time to progression (CMF 5 months, MMM 6 months), or overall survival (CMF 12 months, MMM 16 months). Fifty-two patients received crossover treatment, 48 of whom were evaluable for response. Eight of 23 patients (35%) originally given MMM subsequently responded to crossover treatment with cyclophosphamide/5-FU; 7 had previously responded to MMM. One of 25 patients (4%) originally given CMF subsequently responded to crossover treatment with mitomycin/mitoxantrone; 12 had previously responded to CMF.

Toxicity Results

In general, CMF and MMM were well tolerated, with a low incidence of severe toxicity (WHO grades 3 and 4). Details of subjective toxicity are given in table 2. A significantly higher incidence of diarrhea (all grades) occurred in patients receiving CMF (50%) compared with patients receiving MMM (21%; $p<0.001$); no other significant differences in subjective toxicity were noted. The reduction of 5-FU doses in 3 patients (by 25% in 2, by 75% in 1) resulted in an improvement in symptoms, allowing treatment to continue. As shown in table 2, the incidence of mucositis dropped significantly ($p=0.05$ for CMF; $p=0.02$ for MMM) after the introduction of leucovorin

Table 2. Subjective toxicity (patients with WHO grades 1–4) CMF versus MMM

	CMF		MMM	
WHO Grade	1–2	3–4	1–2	3–4
Alopecia	67	7	58	7
Nausea/vomiting	70	6	62	11
Mucositis				
Before Feb. 1987[1]	63	5	67	–
After Feb. 1987	38	2	33	2
Diarrhea*	43	7	19	2
Lethargy	19	2	16	–
Infection	8	3	18	3

From Jodrell et al. [15], with permission.
* $p<0.001$ (Mann-Whitney test).
1 Prophylactic leucovorin commenced Feb. 1987.

Table 3. Hematologic toxicity (% patients): CMF versus MMM

	WHO Grade			
	1	2	3	4
Anemia[1]				
CMF	25	20	4	–
MMM	30	28	5	–
Leukopenia[1]				
CMF	25	29	15	7
MMM	19	32	23	2
Thrombocytopenia*				
CMF	5	–	5	4
MMM	9	11	9	5

* $p= 0.03$.
1 Not significant.

rescue. Significant alopecia requiring a wig was uncommon, occurring in only 7% of patients in each treatment group.

Hematologic Toxicity. Hematologic toxicity leading to delays in treatment and/or greater than 25% dose reductions occurred in 15 and 20% of patients treated with CMF (total 35%) and 18 and 21% treated with MMM (total 43%), respectively (difference not significant, $p=0.2$). Details are shown in table 3. Thrombocytopenia ($<100\times10^9$/l) occurred in a total of 34% of patients receiving MMM and 14% receiving CMF, and this difference is significant at the 5% level. WHO grades 3 or 4 leukopenia (WBC count $<2.0\times10^9$/l) occurred in 25% of patients receiving MMM and 22% receiving CMF. There was 1 death associated with leukopenia in a patient receiving CMF.

Cardiotoxicity. Of the 75 patients who commenced the cardiac scan protocol, only 45 (60%) had a second, post-initial treatment scan. The reasons for the failure to complete these studies included poor clinical condition (27% of patients), refusal (3%), depression (1%), chest well radiotherapy (3%), and difficulty traveling (7%). Six of 45 patients (13%) were noted to have a significant reduction (>10%) in LVEF after initial treatment. Surprisingly, 4 of these patients had been treated with CMF. One of 2 patients with reduction in LVEF while receiving MMM had an abnormal ECG at the start of treatment (left axis deviation), and neither patient suffered symptoms of cardiac failure. Histologic examination of myocardial tissue was not undertaken.

Trial 2: MMM Versus VAC

Patient Characteristics

Two hundred seventeen patients with histologically or cytologically confirmed breast cancer were entered into this study at the Sutton branch of the Royal Marsden Hospital Breast Unit. Patients were ineligible if they had received prior chemotherapy either as adjuvant treatment or for advanced disease. Patients with significant nonmetastatic cardiac, renal, or hepatic dysfunction were excluded from the study. Details of patient characteristics are given in table 4. After exclusions because of protocol violation, 106 patients were randomized to receive MMM and 105 patients to VAC chemotherapy. Median patient age was 55 and 58 years for patients in the MMM and VAC groups, respectively.

Treatment

Patients were randomized to receive one of the following two schedules: MMM-mitomycin 7 mg/m^2 i.v. every 6 weeks; mitoxantrone 7 mg/m^2 i.v. every 3 weeks; methotrexate 35 mg/m^2 i.v. every 3 weeks (maximum dose, 50 mg). VAC – vincristine 1.4 mg/m^2 every 3 weeks (maximum dose, 2 mg); anthracycline (doxorubicin or epirubicin) 30 mg/m^2 every 3 weeks; cyclophosphamide 400 mg/m^2 every 3 weeks. Both treatments were usually given on an outpatient basis. Choice of doxorubicin or epirubicin for patients receiving VAC was made in a double-blind randomization. All patients received antiemetic prophylaxis, usually with metoclopramide 20 mg i.v. and

Table 4. Patient characteristics: MMM versus VAC

	MMM	VAC
Patients, n	107	110
Exclusions because of previous chemotherapy	1	5
Included in analysis	106	105
Median age, years (range)	55 (36–77)	58 (30–76)
Menopausal status		
Pre	15	15
Post	83	80
Peri	4	5
Unknown	3	4
Previous treatment		
Adjuvant endocrine	23	26
Adjuvant chemotherapy	0	0
Endocrine for advanced disease (responders)	71 (27)	73 (32)
Sites of disease, n		
Local	47	50
Skin	9	10
Nodes	41	24
Lung	35	40
Liver	31	34
Bone	59	63
CNS	5	1
Other	32	39
Median interval from diagnosis to first relapse, months (range)	16 (0–15)	15 (0–16)
Median interval from first relapse to start of chemotherapy, months (range)	8 (0–15)	8 (0–8)

From Jodrell et al. [15], with permission.

dexamethasone 8 mg i.v. with chemotherapy, followed by orally administered metoclopramide and dexamethasone for 3–4 days after treatment. All patients receiving VAC were offered scalp cooling with chemotherapy, providing they had adequate liver function. Treatment was continued for at least 6 courses in patients achieving an objective response (symptomatic relief). Since our trial of MMM versus CMF had initially shown an unacceptable incidence of troublesome mucositis, leucovorin rescue was given to all patients in this trial as a safeguard.

Assessment of Response and Toxicity

Details are the same as those cited in the trial of MMM versus CMF.

Response Results

A total of 189 patients were evaluable for response; the remainder were excluded because of early deaths or inadequate follow-up. There was no significant difference between treatment groups in the overall response rate, which was 53% (96 patients) for MMM (95% CI, 43–62%) and 49% (93 patients) for VAC (95% CI, 39–58%). Six patients in each arm achieved a CR. Response rate by site of metastatic disease was similar for both arms. There was no significant difference between treatment groups in median response duration, which was 10 and 11 months for MMM and VAC, respectively. Similarly, there was no significant difference in median survival, which was 8 months for patients receiving MMM and 10 months for patients receiving VAC.

Toxicity Results

Details regarding nonhematologic and hematologic toxicity are given in tables 5 and 6, respectively. The main differences between treatment groups were a lack of significant neuropathy ($p<0.001$) and of severe alopecia ($p<0.001$) among patients receiving MMM. Likewise, the severity of nausea and vomiting was significantly less in patients receiving MMM. In terms of hematologic toxicity, the trend toward myelosuppression was greater in the MMM arm than in the VAC arm ($p<0.001$). Systemic infection related to myelosuppression and requiring parenteral antibiotics occurred in 2 patients receiving MMM and in 5 receiving VAC. There were no treatment-related deaths.

Discussion

Combination chemotherapy achieves response rates of approximately 50 to 60% in patients with metastatic breast cancer [7–9] but it has proved difficult to demonstrate a significant survival benefit with currently available drugs [10]. One of the key aims of treatment, therefore, is symptom palliation. It is important that new treatments are not merely active but are also well tolerated. These trials indicate that MMM is an active, well-tolerated chemotherapy regimen with efficacy very similar to that of standard CMF or VAC regimens. In terms of toxicity, MMM is similar to CMF and less toxic than VAC. In particular, severe alopecia was rare using MMM. It must be noted that although MMM use was associated with a low incidence of severe subjective toxicity, significant hematologic toxicity occurred, particularly with the slightly larger total dose used in the first trial (against CMF). In

Table 5. Patients experiencing non-hematologic toxicity: MMM versus VAC (WHO grades 0–4)

	MMM				VAC			
WHO Grade	0	1	2	3–4	0	1	2	3–4
Alopecia*	64 (65)	28 (28)	5 (5)	2 (2)	26 (31)	13 (15)	17 (20)	29 (34)
Neuropathy*	95 (95)	3 (3)	1 (1)		49 (58)	20 (24)	12 (14)	4 (5)
Stomatitis[1]	70 (70)	18 (18)	9 (9)	1 (1)	63 (74)	12 (14)	9 (11)	1 (1)
Nausea+	470 (75)	97 (15)	52 (8)	8 (1)	326 (67)	104 (22)	43 (9)	10 (2)
Vomiting*	558 (89)	39 (6)	25 (4)	4 (1)	393 (81)	61 (13)	22 (5)	8 (2)

* $p<0.001$. Values in parentheses are percentages.
+ $p<0.01$. Numbers for nausea and vomiting represent individual episodes (> 1/pt); values in parentheses are percentages.
1 Not significant.

Table 6. Hematologic toxicity expressed as number of courses as measured at the time of next treatment (i.e., Day 21)

Group	Total courses	Courses, n WHO Grade			
		0	1	2	3
Anemia*, g/dl:		≥11.0	9.5–10.9	8.0–9.4	≤7.9
MMM+	519	371 (71)	120 (23)	24 (5)	4 (1)
VAC	429	350 (82)	61 (14)	16 (4)	2 (1)
Leukopenia*, × 10^9/l:		≥4.0	3.9–3.9	2.0–2.9	≤1.9
MMM	519	322 (62)	114 (22)	68 (13)	15 (3)
VAC	429	333 (77)	68 (16)	27 (6)	1 (1)
Thrombocytopenia*, × 10^9/l:		≥100	75–99	50–74	≤50
MMM	519	495 (95)	8 (2)	9 (2)	7 (1)
VAC	429	427 (99)	1 (<1)	1 (<1)	0 (0)

* $p<0.01$.
+ 110 patients received VAC; 107 patients received MMM.
Values in parentheses are percentages.

that trial 43% of patients required treatment delay or dose reduction. In particular, MMM was more likely than CMF to cause thrombocytopenia (34 vs. 14% of patients, respectively, $p=0.03$).

The results of our cardiotoxicity study were unexpected. Mitoxantrone has established clinical toxicity [11–13], although the drug appears significantly less cardiotoxic than other anthracyclines [12]. In the absence of predisposing factors, mitoxantrone-induced cardiotoxicity is unusual at cumulative doses up to 160 mg/m^2 [14], which is well above the cumulative dose we used (48 mg/m^2 after 6 courses). No evidence of cardiac failure was seen in this study. Four of 6 patients who had significant reductions in LVEF turned out to have been treated with CMF rather than MMM. This suggests that deteriorating cardiac function may relate to advanced metastatic cancer rather than directly to therapies, and casts doubt on studies alleging mitoxantrone- and anthracycline-related cardiotoxicity.

In conclusion, these trials indicate that MMM is an effective regimen for first-line palliative chemotherapy in patients with advanced breast cancer, with advantages over doxorubicin-containing regimens. We feel that it is suitable for study in adjuvant therapy or primary medical therapy of breast cancer.

Acknowledgment

We wish to thank Mrs. Julia Holborn for her help in preparing this manuscript.

References

1 Van Oosterom AT, Powles TJ, Hamersma E, et al: A phase II study of mitomycin C in refractory advanced breast cancer. A multi-centre pilot study; in Mouridsen HT, Palsof T (eds): Breast Cancer – Experimental & Clinical Aspects. Proc 2nd EORTC Breast Cancer Conference, Copenhagen, 1979. Copenhagen, Pergamon Press, 1979, pp 275–276.

2 Stuart-Harris RC, Bozek T, Pavlidis NA, et al: Mitoxantrone: An active new agent in the treatment of advanced breast cancer. Cancer Chemother Pharmacol 1984;12:1–4.

3 Hayward JL, Carbone PP, Heuson J-C, et al: Assessment of response to therapy in advanced breast cancer. Eur J Cancer 1977;13:89–94.

4 Peto R, Pike MC, Armitage P, et al: Design and analysis of randomised clinical trials requiring prolonged observation of each patient. Part 2. Analysis and examples. Br J Cancer 1977;35:1–39.

5 WHO Handbook on Reporting Results of Cancer Treatment. Geneva, WHO Offset Publication No. 48, 1979.

6 Kennedy JW, Sorensen SG, Ritchie JL, et al: Radionuclide angiography for the evaluation of anthracycline therapy. Cancer Treat Rep 1978;62:941–943.

7 Cummings FJ, Gelman R, Horton J: Comparison of CAF versus CMFP in metastatic breast cancer: Analysis of prognostic factors. J Clin Oncol 1985;3:932–940.

8 Aisner J, Weinberg L, Perloff M, et al: Chemotherapy versus chemoimmunotherapy (CAF v CAFVP v CMF each ± MER) for metastatic carcinoma of the breast: A CALGB study. J Clin Oncol 1987;5:1523–1533.

9 Coates A, Gebski V, Bishop J, et al: Improving the quality of life during chemotherapy for advanced breast cancer. N Engl J Med 1987;317;1490–1495.

10 Powles TJ, Smith IE, Ford HT, et al: Failure of chemotherapy to prolong survival in a group of patients with metastatic breast cancer. Lancet 1980;i:580–582.

11 Benjamin RS, Chawla SP, Ewer MS, et al: Evaluation of mitoxantrone cardiac toxicity by nuclear angiography and endomyocardial biopsy: An update. Invest New Drugs 1985;3:117–121.

12 Henderson CI, Allegra JC, Woodcock T, et al: Randomized clinical trial comparing mitoxantrone with doxorubicin in previously treated patients with metastatic breast cancer. J Clin Oncol 1989;7:560–571.

13 Stuart-Harris RC, Pearson M, Smith IE, et al: Cardiotoxicity associated with mitoxantrone. Lancet 1984;ii: 219–220.

14 Posner LE, Dukart G, Goldberg J, et al: Mitoxantrone: An overview of safety and toxicity. Invest New Drugs 1985;3:123–132.

15 Jodrell DI, Smith IE, Mansi JL, et al: A randomised comparative trial of mitoxantrone/methotrexate/mitomycin C (MMM) and cyclophosphamide/methotrexate/5FU (CMF) in the treatment of advanced breast cancer. Br J Cancer 1991;63:794–798.

Oncology 1993;50(suppl 1):16–23

Scot M. Sedlacek

Rose Breast Center,
Rose Medical Center, Denver, Colo., USA

First-Line and Salvage Therapy of Metastatic Breast Cancer with Mitomycin/Vinblastine

Key Words
Mitomycin
Salvage therapy
First-line therapy
Metastatic breast cancer

Abstract
The combination chemotherapy regimen of mitomycin/vinblastine has been used in the treatment of metastatic breast cancer since the early 1980s. We report results of use of mitomycin/vinblastine in 35 women with metastatic breast cancer who had failed prior treatment with one to four chemotherapeutic regimens. Despite heavy prior treatment and significant tumor burdens, 34% of patients achieved a partial remission and another 14% had disease stabilization with a very acceptable toxicity profile. This regimen was also used for the first time as first-line chemotherapy in 11 women with metastatic breast cancer. Response was observed in 9 of 11 patients (82%). Hemolytic-uremic syndrome occurred in 6 of the 46 women (13%) treated in the two protocols and is the most serious potential complication. Mitomycin/vinblastine is an effective salvage regimen and an excellent first-line chemotherapeutic treatment for women with metastatic breast cancer.

Over the past 30 years, cytotoxic chemotherapeutic agents have become the mainstay of treatment for recurrent/metastatic breast cancer. Despite the discovery and use of newer drugs and multidrug regimens, however, we have been unable to achieve a meaningful prolongation of median survival in women with metastatic breast cancer beyond that seen with additive or ablative hormone therapy or even no therapy at all [1, 2]. Indeed, some investigators have reported that women receiving cytotoxic chemotherapy died sooner than the average untreated woman with recurrent/metastatic breast cancer, who lives approximately 18–24 months [3]. As the concept of dose intensity became popular, results obtained with various chemotherapeutic regimens were compared [4], and it became clear that the more dose-intensive a schedule for a particular regimen, the higher objective response rate achieved. Unfortunately, despite tremendous differences in dose intensity (and, therefore, response rates), there were no significant differences in overall survival rates.

Since we have been unable to cure or even significantly prolong the lives of women with metastatic breast cancer, our primary goal has been palliation of disease symptoms. To relieve pain from bony metastases, shortness of breath from lung or pleural tumor involvement, or cachexia and fatigue from liver metastases, one must reduce the tumor volume or obtain an objective response (partial or complete response, PR or CR). For the patient with seemingly unrelenting disease progression, the ability to halt progression may provide a meaningful benefit (stabilization). Because the agents used to obtain these benefits also carry the potential for significant toxicity and side effects, a balance must be struck between 'pushing' regimens to

Scot M. Sedlacek, MD
4500 E Ninth Avenue
Suite 140
Denver, CO 80220 (USA)

0030–2414/93/0507–0016
$2.75/0

obtain a response and causing so many toxic side effects that overall palliation is negated [5]. The treatment should not be worse than the cancer itself. With this in mind, we studied the efficacy and safety of combination mitomycin/vinblastine in the first-line salvage treatment of women with metastatic breast cancer.

Mitomycin/Vinblastine: Dosing

The initial dosage of mitomycin used in this study was 10 mg/m^2 every 4 weeks. The initial dosage of vinblastine was 6 mg/m^2 i.v. every 2 weeks. Patients who lived a great distance from Denver received vinblastine 6 mg/m^2 on a 4-week basis along with the mitomycin. Cognizant of this regimen's myelosuppressive effects, we decreased doses and/or prolonged the dosing interval in an attempt to minimize complications from significant neutropenia and/or thrombocytopenia.

Use as Salvage Therapy

Patient Characteristics

The median age of the 35 women given mitomycin/vinblastine as salvage therapy was 50 years (range, 32–72). In addition to treatment with mitomycin/vinblastine, 12 women received adjuvant chemotherapy with mainly CMF (cyclophosphamide/methotrexate/5-fluorouracil, 5-FU)-based regimens (table 1); 1 patient received doxorubicin. Previous therapy consisted of a mean of 1.5 chemotherapy regimens (range, 1–4) (table 2) and 1.3 hormone regimens (range, 0–4) (table 3). Thus, mitomycin/vinblastine represented the fourth line of therapy in the metastatic setting. Twenty-two patients who had previously received anthracyclines eventually developed resistance to these agents as manifested by disease progression. These women displayed fairly extensive disease involvement, with an average of 2.5 metastatic sites per patient (range, 1–6). Sites included bone, lung, liver, bone marrow, and soft tissue (table 4).

Table 1. Adjuvant chemotherapy (n = 12)

Regimen	Patients, n
CMFT	8
CMFVP	3
AC	1

CMFT = cyclophosphamide/methotrexate/5-FU/tamoxifen; CMFVP = cyclophosphamide/methotrexate/5-FU/vincristine/prednisone; AC = doxorubicin/cyclophosphamide.

Table 2. Previous chemotherapy (n = 35)[1]

Regimen	Patients, n
Anthracyclines	22
CMF/CMFVP	21
CAF	12
Doxorubicin ± vincristine	8
Epirubicin	2
Other	5

CMF = Cyclophosphamide/methotrexate/5-FU; CMFVP = cyclophosphamide/methotrexate/5-FU/vincristine/prednisone; CAF = cyclophosphamide/doxorubicin/5-FU.

[1] Mean 1.5 regimens per patient (range, 1–4).

Table 3. Previous hormone therapy (n = 24)[1]

	Patients, n
Tamoxifen	21
Megestrol acetate	13
Aminoglutethimide/hydrocortisone	6
Oophorectomy	2
Tamoxifen/megestrol acetate	1
Halotestin	1
Diethylstilbestrol	1

[1] Mean 1.3 regimens per patient (range, 0–4).

Results

Of the 35 patients treated with the mitomycin/vinblastine salvage regimen, 12 (34%) obtained an objective PR; there were no CRs. This fourth-line salvage regimen may have benefited as many as 17 women (49%) however; an additional 5 (14%) showed stabilization of disease progression. Eighteen patients (51%) had progressive disease. Categorizing patients by the number of previously received chemotherapeutic regimens for metastatic disease revealed that 9 of 23 patients (39%) obtained a PR when mitomycin/vinblastine was used as second-line chemotherapy, and 3 of 12 (25%) obtained a PR when it was used as third-, fourth-, or fifth-line chemotherapy. Among women resistant to previous treatment with anthracyclines, 6 of 22 (27%) obtained an objective re-

Table 4. Sites of disease (n = 35)[1]

Site	Patients, n
Bone	22
Skin	14
Lung	11
Pleura	11
Liver	10
Lymph nodes	10
Bone marrow	3
CNS	3
Pericardium	2
Retina	1

[1] Mean 2.5 sites per patient (range, 1–6).

Table 5. Sites of response (n = 35)

Site	Responses, n
Bone	0/22
Skin	3/14
Lung	6/11
Liver	3/10
Lymph nodes	2/10
Bone marrow	1/3

sponse, with another 2 (9%) achieving stabilization. On the other hand, 6 of 13 women (46%) who had not received prior treatment with anthracyclines responded to mitomycin/vinblastine, with an additional 3 (23%) achieving stabilization.

Despite the great difficulty in obtaining a 50% reduction of tumor in bony sites, many patients with such metastases in this study reported subjective improvement in bone pain, with a resultant decreased requirement for narcotic pain medications. In sites where disease was measurable, responses were observed in tumors of the lung, liver, lymph nodes, and skin (table 5).

The median number of cycles of mitomycin/vinblastine received was 3 (range, 1–11). The median duration of response was 5 months (range, 3–41). One of the most interesting and potentially clinically important observations made in this trial was that the median rapidity of response was 3 weeks (range, 2–8). Had patients been assessed more frequently, responses might have been recorded even sooner.

From the time we initiated therapy, mean survival was about 7.6 months (range 0.1–45). A total of 21 patients received further chemotherapy. Two patients responded to a continuous infusion of 5-FU and 1 patient to cisplatin, for a subsequent response rate of 14% (3 of 21). Six patients received subsequent hormone therapy, but no objective responses were observed.

Toxicity

Nonhematologic side effects were mild to moderate in severity and usually easily managed. Three episodes of extravasation occurred in 2 patients prior to the use of central venous catheters, which are now routinely employed for the administration of known vesicants. Three women experienced an unusual syndrome of gastrointestinal dysmotility manifested by severe constipation, with nausea and vomiting occurring 4–5 days after each vinblastine dose and lasting 4–6 days. On some occasions this led to hospitalization for dehydration. This condition did not recur upon discontinuation of vinblastine. Two other women complained of grades 1–2 nausea after receiving mitomycin/vinblastine. One patient had significant diffuse arthralgias related to the use of vinblastine. One death occurred in a woman who had received two cycles of mitomycin/vinblastine, achieved a PR, but then discontinued therapy. She developed adult respiratory distress syndrome 2 months after ending treatment and died of respiratory failure. At autopsy, no etiology for this syndrome was identified.

Hematologic toxicity was moderate. The mean nadir WBC count during therapy was 2.3×10^9/l (median, 1.6), and the mean nadir platelet count was 121×10^9/l (median, 76). A total of 15 women required dose reductions and another 13 cycle prolongations due to low WBC and low platelet counts. One patient developed significant anemia requiring RBC transfusions, whereas 2 patients had to be hospitalized for neutropenic fever. Four women ultimately developed hemolytic-uremic syndrome.

Use as First-Line Chemotherapy

Encouraged by the high rate and rapidity of response obtained with mitomycin/vinblastine in salvage therapy, as well as by the combination's favorable toxicity profile, we commenced a study using this regimen for the first time as first-line chemotherapy in patients with metastatic breast cancer.

Patient Characteristics

We initially began selecting patients with massive tumor burdens who required a rapid response, such as those with 80–95% liver replacement with synthetic function compromise and those with lymphatic spread to the lungs requiring supplemental oxygen therapy. We later included women who had refused other chemotherapeutic regimens but who were willing to try mitomycin/vinblastine when told this regimen did not cause alopecia or significant nausea and vomiting. Eleven women with metastatic breast cancer (mean, 2.2 sites; range, 1–5) were treated (table 6). The median patient age was 59 years (range, 36–73). Seven patients had previously received a mean of 1.3 (range, 0–2) hormone regimens for metastatic disease; 9 patients received adjuvant chemotherapy (table 7).

Results

Patients received a median of 4+ cycles of chemotherapy (range, 2–11). Nine women (82%) obtained an objective PR. One patient with lymphatic spread to the lungs had a minor response that stabilized after 3 cycles. Only 1 patient (9%) experienced disease progression, which occurred following 2 cycles of treatment. She had extensive recurrent disease involving the entire left chest wall and neck, which continued to progress despite subsequent administration of radiation therapy to the affected areas. Median rapidity of response (5 weeks; range, 2 weeks to 9 months) was again noted to be of fairly short duration. One patient had a pleural effusion that initially stabilized while she was receiving therapy and required no further thoracenteses. After 9 months of treatment, the effusion finally regressed. She received 11 cycles of mitomycin/vinblastine before going on a 'drug holiday', which lasted 8 months. Median duration of response was 5+ months (range, 1+ to 9+). Despite extensive visceral involvement, 4 of 5 patients with lung involvement and all 4 patients with liver involvement demonstrated objective disease regression.

Toxicity

The mitomycin/vinblastine regimen was as well tolerated in first-line treatment as it was in salvage therapy. One patient each had chemical phlebitis and extravasation. One patient developed vinblastine-associated dysmotility syndrome, which ceased upon discontinuation of vinblastine. One woman with extensive liver replacement experienced moderate alopecia, which resolved as her disease regressed and despite continued treatment.

Hematologic toxicity is the most common and significant side effect noted with this regimen (table 8). Two patients developed symptomatic anemia requiring packed RBC transfusions and 2 patients developed hemolytic-uremic syndrome. Despite all 11 women requiring a dose reduction and/or cycle prolongation due to a low WBC count, only 1 patient after 1 cycle developed neutropenic fever.

Table 6. Sites of disease (n = 11)[1]

Site	Patients, n
Bone	6
Lung	5
Liver	4
Chest wall	3
Retina	2
Brain	1
Pleura	1
Pericardium	1
Lymph nodes	1

[1] Mean 2.2 sites per patient (range, 1–5).

Table 7. Previous treatment (n = 11)

	Patients, n
Hormonal therapy[1]	7
Adjuvant chemotherapy	9
CMF	7
CMF/CAF	1
Thiotepa	1

CMF = Cyclophosphamide/methotrexate/5-FU; CAF = cyclophosphamide/doxorubicin/5-FU.
[1] Mean 1.3 regimens per patient (range, 0–2).

Hemolytic-Uremic Syndrome

Hemolytic-uremic syndrome developed in 2 of 11 women (18%) receiving mitomycin/vinblastine as first-line treatment and in 4 of 35 (11%) given the regimen as salvage therapy. A total of 6 of 46 patients (13%) therefore developed this syndrome. Patients remained free of hemolytic-uremic syndrome during cycles 1–3; it developed in 2 patients following cycle 4, in 2 patients following cycle 5, and in 1 each following cycles 6 and 7. A total of 164 cycles

Table 8. Hematologic toxicity

Nadir[1] WBC count × 10⁹/l	Nadir[1] platelet count, × 10⁹/l	Dose reduction	Cycle prolongation	Due to low platelet count	Due to low WBC count	Hemolytic-uremic syndrome	RBC transfusion
0.9	18	+	+	+	+	+	
3.0	109	+	+	+	+		+
2.4	78	+			+		
2.7	136		+		+		
1.1	15	+	+	+	+		
2.0	73	+		+	+		
1.0	228	+	+		+		
2.3	267	+	+		+		
2.0	21	+	+	+	+		
2.0	58	+	+	+	+		+
1.3	231	+			+	+	
2.0	78						

1 Median.

Table 9. Hemolytic-uremic syndrome

Patient No.	Staph A pheresis	HUS response	Cancer response	Duration of response, months	Follow-up	Cause of death
28	Yes	No	No	–	Died, 4 days	HUS
38	Yes	Yes	Yes	9	Alive	–
45	Yes	Partial	No	–	Died, 2 months	Cancer
51	Yes	No	No	–	Died, 11 days	Cancer
54	Yes	Partial	No	–	Died, 44 days	Cancer
59	Yes	Yes	Yes	6	Alive, CRF	–

HUS = Hemolytic-uremic syndrome; CRF = chronic renal failure.

of mitomycin/vinblastine were given in the two studies; all 6 cases of hemolytic-uremic syndrome occurred during delivery of the final 51 cycles of treatment, which translates to a 12% incidence for cycles 4–11 and a 4% incidence overall.

All patients with hemolytic-uremic syndrome underwent pheresis over a Prosorba immunoadsorption treatment column (Imré Corporation, Seattle, Wash.) [6, 7]. Two patients experienced complete reversal of the syndrome, while 2 others had partial reversal (table 9). To date, only 1 patient from these studies has died of hemolytic-uremic syndrome.

We retrospectively reviewed patient charts in an attempt to determine whether there was some way of predicting which patients would eventually develop hemolytic-uremic syndrome. We noted that lactate dehydrogenase (LDH) levels rose in all 6 patients with hemolytic-uremic syndrome 1–3 months prior to diagnosis. All of these patients were in continued remission at the time of LDH elevation, thus suggesting that the rise resulted from RBC destruction. Serum creatinine levels rose in 3 of the 6 patients 1–2 months prior to diagnosis; 4 of 6 developed anemia requiring transfusion 1–4 months prior to diagnosis. Five women developed hemolytic-uremic syndrome while actively receiving mitomycin/vinblastine; the 6th developed it 3 months after progressing with mitomycin/vinblastine and while receiving cisplatin, another drug that has been rarely implicated in this syndrome.

Conclusion

The combination of mitomycin/vinblastine is an effective salvage regimen for patients with metastatic breast cancer, including those heavily pretreated and those showing resistance to prior treatment with anthracyclines. When given as first-line chemotherapy, the regimen has demonstrated efficacy even in patients with significant tumor burden. Rapid responses to mitomycin/vinblastine have been shown to occur within the first 2–5 weeks of treatment. Hematologic toxicity, including leukopenia and thrombocytopenia, may require dose reductions and/or cycle prolongations, but is rarely associated with infectious or bleeding complications. Hemolytic-uremic syndrome is the most significant dose-dependent complication observed with mitomycin/vinblastine; in responding patients it may be heralded by a rise in LDH levels.

We recommend using mitomycin/vinblastine as first-line chemotherapy in patients whose cancer requires a rapid response and as salvage therapy in patients with a favorable risk/benefit ratio. Because of the significant risk of hemolytic-uremic syndrome posed after 4 cycles of treatment, however, continued use of this regimen beyond 4 cycles must be viewed with caution, especially in responders who develop elevated LDH levels.

References

1 Patel JK, Nemoto T, Vezeridis M, et al: Does more intense palliative treatment improve overall survival in metastatic breast cancer patients? Cancer 1986;57:567–570.

2 Alexander HG, Paterson MD, Szafran O, et al: Effect of chemotherapy on survival in metastatic breast cancer. Breast Cancer Res Treat 1981;1:357–363.

3 Powles TJ, Smith IE, Ford HT, et al: Failure of chemotherapy to prolong survival in a group of patients with metastatic breast cancer. Lancet 1980;i:580–582.

4 Hryniuk W, Bush H: The importance of dose intensity in chemotherapy of metastatic breast cancer. J Clin Oncol 1984;2:1281–1288.

5 Tannock IF, Boyd NF, DeBoer G, et al: A randomized trial of two dose levels of cyclophosphamide, methotrexate, and fluorouracil chemotherapy for patients with metastatic breast cancer. J Clin Oncol 1988;6:1377–1387.

6 Korec S, Schein PS, Smith FP, et al: Treatment of cancer-associated hemolytic uremic syndrome with staphylococcal protein A immunoperfusion. J Clin Oncol 1986;4:210–215.

7 Snyder H, Mittelman A, Korec S: Protein A immunoadsorption therapy in the treatment of hemolytic uremic syndrome associated with cancer therapy (abstract). Proc Am Soc Clin Oncol 1990;9:320.

Discussion

Dr. Henderson: Mitomycin is clearly among the more effective drugs for the treatment of breast cancer, both as a single agent and in combination with other agents. Yet many of the toxicities associated with mitomycin use – such as the acute pulmonary syndrome that may occur when mitomycin is combined with a vinca alkaloid, pulmonary fibrosis, and particularly hemolytic-uremic syndrome – are not very well studied or very well described. Why have so few studies been done? Why do we have so few data on what appears to be one of the best agents for the treatment of breast cancer?

Dr. Gralla: We really don't even have a handle on this drug in terms of efficacy, where dose dependency is a major consideration, much less toxicity. I believe one of the things that block use of this drug in breast cancer or lung cancer is the clinician's fear of toxicities that have rarely been encountered.

Dr. Henderson: Do you think that was a problem 10 years ago?

Dr. Gralla: I think it was. The drug got a bad reputation early on and was pigeonholed into a category of being active in gastrointestinal malignancies and having few other uses. I think today many clinicians, on encountering unusual toxicities with an unfamiliar drug, will be reluctant to use that drug again. Yet such was not the case with doxorubicin, a drug that was originally linked to cardiotoxicity described as sudden and unpredictable. That certainly did not stop clinicians from using it. Why hasn't this happened with mitomycin?

Dr. Hortobagyi: I would guess because doxorubicin had the advantage of coming along later, and at the same time as other drugs like cisplatin, which had different toxicities. Mitomycin had already come and gone.

Dr. Sedlacek: I think it's also the perceived irreversibility of cumulative hematologic toxicity, or myelosuppression, that has kept people away. Again, in my experience, this toxicity is reversible – the bone marrow does recover. Even the attending physicians I work with who deal with malignancies other than breast cancer are frightened by it, though. But now we have a very effective therapy for the hemolytic-uremic syndrome, staph protein A pheresis. At the last ASCO meeting, one group reported an updated 70% response rate.

Dr. Smith: I think initially the point Dr. Gralla makes is true. The drug started off with a bad reputation. But in the last 10 or 15 years, particularly in breast cancer, no one has been pushing this drug commercially, and I really think that's important. I think the other important thing is that, despite having been on the market for a long time and despite an enormous body of information, there is relatively little useful information about mitomycin, which is probably not true for some of the other drugs that were developed later. The dose question, for example, has not been properly addressed in any disease that I know. The schedule was always developed empirically in trials.

Dr. Schnall: I agree with Dr. Smith. Furthermore, I think we've all been taught that the single best agent for breast cancer is doxorubicin. That's why when treatment fails with, say CMF (cyclophosphamide/methotrexate/5-fluorouracil), you go right to doxorubicin. Rarely does your thought process skip to mitomycin before you hit doxorubicin. So to some degree I think it is marketing, as well as some folklore that has been passed around.

Dr. Keane: I think it's a combination of events. Consider the age distribution of medical oncologists around the world. Many of the people who are in practice today were not around when mitomycin was first introduced and therefore have no personal experience with it. What they have gleaned from the literature is that mitomycin was associated with distressing and perhaps idiosyncratic toxicity. In the absence of personal experience and with alternatives available, it's very easy to say, 'I'm not going to buy into that experience. Why should I?'

This drug has some unique features and really has a role. I think that's what we should focus on in terms of our discussion. What are the arguments that suggest that this drug should be looked at again? Based on what I've heard today, evidence that this drug is very toxic when used in a reasonable way is just not there when you look at the data.

Dr. Henderson: So you would argue that mitomycin's relative lack of toxicity is justification for its use. To that I would add that I think it's one drug for which there's more convincing evidence than any other of a lack of cross-resistance with doxorubicin and cyclophosphamide. That's why I've been fascinated with mitomycin for quite a few years.

Dr. Hortobagyi: One of the things that we found in our randomized trial, and which was mentioned by several speakers here, is that responses to mitomycin occur rather rapidly. Without a comparative trial it's hard to tell whether mitomycin produces responses more rapidly than drug B, C, or D, but certainly the impression I have is that most of the responses occur early, within the first 4–6 weeks. I think this is an advantage, especially for symptomatic patients.

Dr. Henderson: What would be the rationale for studying this drug further? Or, to put it another way, what do you think are the highest priority studies that should be performed?

Dr. Smith: One issue that deserves further study is dose rate. I'm not advocating doing studies using high-dose schedules with bone marrow rescue. I'm talking about something quite simple, say 10 mg/m^2 every 4 weeks versus 8 mg/m^2 every 6 weeks.

Dr. Henderson: You'd look at those doses using mitomycin as a single agent?

Dr. Smith: That's one of the problems. Here's a drug that is active in second-line treatment, perhaps highly active in first-line treatment, with very little subjective toxicity. There's no doubt if mitomycin was a new phase II drug that was just beginning to be evaluated in the treatment of breast cancer, we'd be really excited. But the drug has been around a long time.

Dr. Henderson: Of course, there are also plenty of funds available to support studies with new agents, which isn't an unimportant point.

Dr. Smith: That's right. But I think certainly one question that needs addressing is, what's the best way of scheduling this drug?

Dr. Gralla: I think that everyone around this table is convinced that mitomycin has activity, even though there's a paucity of single-agent studies. Yet, if toxicities are greater when mitomycin is combined with a vinca alkaloid in the treatment of breast cancer, for instance, additional single-agent studies may be very important, because there may be less toxicity, especially in the palliative area. I could see using different schedules of an extremely low dose combined with other agents versus moderate and slightly higher single-agent doses, say 4–5 mg/m^2 and 8–10 mg/m^2, in previously treated or untreated patients. I think we have to ask ourselves what the end points will be. Response rate and toxicity would be easy to show, but survival may be extraordinarily difficult and require a huge study in order to compile convincing data.

Dr. Henderson: One thing I have repeatedly heard in this symposium is that current data are insufficient to substantiate the claim that mitomycin is more effective when combined with a vinca alkaloid or any other agent than when used alone. This is presumably an issue some might find worthwhile studying.

Dr. Smith: That clearly needs to be addressed. I also think the data presented today are compelling enough to pursue additional studies in previously untreated patients. I'm not terribly excited about the concept of studying mitomycin as a single agent, but acknowledge some single-agent studies might need to be done. Additionally, we need to explore the drug in other combinations. A number of drugs that are effective in breast cancer have less overlapping toxicity with mitomycin – 5-FU by continuous infusion, for example, can be combined with this agent very well, which would allow for the addition of other myelosuppressive drugs.

Dr. Gralla: The third reason, then, for studying this agent is that it is easy to use in combination with a variety of other active agents. We've also said that it has a seemingly relatively low toxicity pattern, depending, of course, on dose and schedule. And it has an apparently unique mechanism of action with lack of cross-resistance.

Dr. Henderson: I'd like to throw out one last provocative question. In the recent approval of granulocyte colony-stimulating factor (G-CSF), the US Food and Drug Administration specifically mentioned mitomycin as a drug that has not yet been used (or at least studied) in combination with G-CSF. Nevertheless, it seems plausible that the use of G-CSF with mitomycin will circumvent one of its major toxicities – prolonged myelosuppression. Future use of peripheral blood progenitor cells will probably be effective in circumventing thrombocytopenia, at least until we have specific growth factors for platelets. Do you think that both of these approaches, one circumventing myelosuppression and one circumventing thrombocytopenia, stand to enhance mitomycin's efficacy by permitting higher doses or a longer duration of therapy to be given?

Dr. Hortobagyi: I think mitomycin's major hematologic toxicity is thrombocytopenia. Neutropenia is seldom, if ever, an issue. So G-CSF or granulocyte macrophage colony-stimulating factor is probably not going to be very useful. Interleukin 3 might be. It's already in clinical trials. I doubt you will need peripheral stem cells for every patient. But they might prove helpful in some patients, especially if subsequent trials show a reason to give mitomycin on a long-term basis, or for more than just a limited number of cycles.

Dr. Henderson: Any other comments?

Dr. Smith: The more I hear, the more I think there may be reason to go back and start phase II studies using this drug as a single agent in previously untreated patients with breast cancer. I think there would be a lot of clinical opportunities for doing this, and we could get data quickly.

Oncology 1993;50(suppl 1):24–30

Robert S. Folman

Department of Medicine, Section of Oncology, Bridgeport Hospital, Bridgeport, Conn., USA

Experience with Mitomycin in the Treatment of Non-Small Cell Lung Cancer

Key Words
Mitomycin
NSCLC
MVP
Vinca alkaloid
Cisplatin
Dose-intensive
Stage IIIA

Abstract
Mitomycin has proven to be among the most active drugs available for the single-agent treatment of non-small cell lung cancer (NSCLC). In combination with vinca alkaloids and cisplatin, mitomycin can produce response rates greater than or equal to 50% in properly selected patients. In our experience, such responses were achieved using moderate doses (7 or 8 mg/m^2) of mitomycin, which also resulted in fewer hematologic and other toxicities. Delivery of MVP (mitomycin/vinca alkaloid/cisplatin) to 150 patients with stages III and IV NSCLC during the last decade showed maximal response was achieved after two or three cycles of therapy. A comparative analysis of results reported using MVP regimens suggests that high response rates are associated with greater dose-intensive use of cisplatin and lesser dose-intensive use of mitomycin. Although the role of MVP in the treatment of advanced NSCLC is unclear, use of mitomycin-containing regimens as part of a multidisciplinary approach to stage IIIA NSCLC has yielded high response rates and has successfully downstaged patients prior to surgery. Randomized clinical trials will be required to validate these findings, but the focus of future research should be on discovering new agents with greater activity and on developing new approaches wherein these agents can be delivered with maximum efficacy and minimum toxicity.

Mitomycin, an antibiotic isolated from *Streptomyces caespitosus,* has proven useful in the treatment of a variety of cancers. Results of single-agent trials indicate that mitomycin is among the most active drugs available for the treatment of non-small cell lung cancer (NSCLC) (table 1) [1–3]. In 1977, Eagan et al. [4] initiated the use of platinum-based polychemotherapy in patients with NSCLC and reported a 39% overall response to the CAP combination (cyclophosphamide/doxorubicin/cisplatin). It is now widely accepted that platinum-based drug combinations offer the best chance of remission for patients with advanced NSCLC. In 1981, Gralla et al. [5] reported a 42% response rate to the combination of vindesine (a vinca alkaloid) and cisplatin. In a later report, Gralla et al. [6] suggested that adding mitomycin to this combination results in even greater efficacy.

During the past decade several large randomized phase III trials have compared the best available drug regimens in advanced NSCLC [7–9]. These trials failed to identify any drug combination or single agent that offers a

Robert S. Folman, MD
15 Corporate Drive
Trumbull, CT 06611 (USA)

0030–2414/93/0507–0024
$2.75/0

major survival advantage over the others tested. Indeed, the very role of chemotherapy in this disease remains a topic of continued discussion and debate [10]. This report will review some of the more important clinical trials involving mitomycin. It will also review our experience with this agent over more than a decade of use in a community oncology practice. It is hoped that this review will help clarify the role of mitomycin and suggest guidelines for its use in NSCLC.

Community Experience with Mitomycin

Oncology Associates of Bridgeport, Conn., is a subspecialty group practice that services the medical oncology needs of Bridgeport Hospital, a 600-bed Yale-affiliated community hospital. In late 1981, after seeing several patients with advanced NSCLC respond to MVP (mitomycin/vinblastine/cisplatin), we undertook a study of that combination in our practice. Prior to that time, we had acquired considerable experience with mitomycin, primarily in combination with 5-fluorouracil (5-FU), or with 5-FU/doxorubicin (FAM), in treating gastrointestinal cancer, and also in breast cancer, and as a single agent in treating NSCLC. In those trials we observed mitomycin-induced lung toxicity, protracted thrombocytopenia, drug extravasation, and 1 tragic case of fatal hemolytic-uremic syndrome in a young patient with colon carcinoma. We therefore commenced our study with a keen awareness of the potential toxicities of mitomycin.

During the past decade we have treated approximately 150 NSCLC patients with MVP. While the vast majority of these patients had stage IIIB or IV disease, we also gave the combination as part of neoadjuvant therapy to patients with stage IIIA disease and as adjuvant chemotherapy to a few patients with resected stage II or IIIA disease. Only a small percentage of the patients received more than four cycles of MVP. Maximal response was generally achieved after two or three cycles of therapy. Radiation therapy was then offered to eligible patients. Our early experience with MVP has been reported previously [11] and will be briefly summarized here.

Fifty-six patients with advanced NSCLC and a Karnofsky performance status of 60 or greater were treated with a regimen consisting of mitomycin 10 mg/m^2 and cisplatin 100 mg/m^2 on day 1, and vinblastine 6 mg/m^2 on day 1 and then every 2 weeks. Treatment was recycled on day 29 and every 6 weeks thereafter. We observed a major overall response of 73%. However, as table 2 [11] illustrates, our early experience with highly selected patients (and good luck) probably biased the study results. A recent chart review of 50 patients treated with MVP during the past 5 years confirms the results observed later in our study and suggests that a 50% response rate can be expected in patients with good performance status.

Table 1. Single-agent activity in patients with NSCLC

	Patients, n	Response, %
Most active agents		
Cisplatin	305	16
Ifosfamide	130	27
Mitomycin	88	17
Vindesine	370	17
Vinblastine	22	27
Etoposide	–	18
Less active agents		
Cyclophosphamide	405	12
Lomustine	216	10
Doxorubicin	296	12
Carboplatin	158	12
5-Fluorouracil	26	8
Methotrexate	105	11

Adapted from Kris et al. [1], Bonomi [2], and Bakowski and Creech [3].

Table 2. MVP in patients with NSCLC (Bridgeport Hospital)

	Responders	
	n	%
1981–1984 (using mitomycin 10 mg/m^2)		
First 18 patients (highly selected)	16	89
Next 34 patients (less selected)	18	53
Total (52 patients)	34	73
1985–1990 (using mitomycin 7–8 mg/m^2)		
50 patients (random chart review)	24	48

Adapted from Folman and Rosman [11].

Lessons from the Community Experience

We have learned several lessons about mitomycin from this experience. First, a good response rate (50%) can be achieved with moderate doses of mitomycin. Several patients in our original series, and all patients treated since the study's conclusion in 1984, have received only 7–8 mg/m^2 per dose of mitomycin without altering the response rate. This finding has been corroborated by Gralla et al. [6, 12] in their extensive experience with mitomycin at the Memorial Sloan-Kettering Cancer Center (MSKCC).

Using low individual and cumulative doses of mitomycin, we rarely encountered serious lasting sequelae from therapy. Two patients developed pulmonary toxicity (interstitial lung infiltrates). There have been no cases of either hemolytic-uremic syndrome or serious renal dysfunction. None of our patients has had protracted thrombocytopenia, although a few developed this problem after radiation therapy was initiated following MVP. Observed myelosuppression was seldom life-threatening. No toxic deaths and few septic hospital admissions have occurred among patients receiving the lower mitomycin dose. Steroids may have played a protective role in reducing some potential toxicities, as all patients received 20–30 mg of dexamethasone on the days of mitomycin/cisplatin therapy.

We also learned that some patients may experience gratifying unmaintained remissions after only two cycles of MVP. The role of maintenance chemotherapy in patients with advanced NSCLC is unknown. Considering the toxicity of high-dose cisplatin therapy, however, we believe maintenance chemotherapy should be avoided, when possible, or given infrequently.

We have not observed significant responses in previously irradiated areas. We have seen, however, regression of asymptomatic brain metastases with chemotherapy alone administered prior to the initiation of radiation therapy. We have observed a few remarkable remissions in patients with poor performance status, but due to poor tolerance and a low probability of benefit, we do not encourage patients with a Karnofsky performance status <80 to undergo therapy. We have been discouraged by the poor survival of even our responding patients treated with MVP (median, 10 months vs. 4 months for nonresponders). However, since patients with advanced NSCLC often desire therapy, and since they improve both subjectively and objectively with a good response to treatment, it remains appropriate to offer them the option of chemotherapy. The MVP combination is certainly among the most active regimens available to oncologists today. The focus of clinical research, however, must be on the discovery of better drugs and more effective combinations. We must also improve our ability to minimize toxicity.

Clinical Trials in Advanced NSCLC

Numerous randomized and nonrandomized clinical trials have attempted to identify the most effective chemotherapy program for NSCLC and to clarify whether and when such therapy should be given to patients outside of a clinical trial. Unfortunately, reviewing these studies one can only draw the following conclusions: (1) There is no single 'best' chemotherapy for NSCLC. (2) Chemotherapy may prolong survival in responding patients but has little impact on overall survival in studies of advanced NSCLC. (3) Patients treated in single-institution studies fare much better than those treated in multi-institution phase III trials (clearly, differences in doses administered and the condition of patients treated must account for the inconsistent outcomes reported by these trials).

The most encouraging reports on the role of mitomycin in NSCLC have come from the MSKCC. Gralla et al. [6] studied the effect of adding mitomycin to the combination of vindesine and cisplatin. In a randomized study of 120 patients with advanced NSCLC, they found that the 3-drug combination (using 120 mg/m^2 of cisplatin) induced a higher response rate than the two-drug combination (54% vs. 39%, $p<0.02$). This response was similar to that seen in our community practice where vinblastine was used instead of vindesine. Indeed, the same investigators have proved that substitution of vinblastine for vindesine can be made without altering response [12]. Mitomycin alone has been compared with the MVP regimen, and the superiority of the combination has been established [13].

Mitomycin has been tested in several phase III multi-institutional clinical trials with disappointing results. In the Eastern Cooperative Oncology Group (ECOG) study of the four most active regimens in metastatic NSCLC [7], an MVP regimen using 10 mg/m^2 of mitomycin and only 40 mg/m^2 of cisplatin was compared with vindesine/cisplatin (120 mg/m^2), etoposide/cisplatin (60 mg/m^2), and a nonplatinum regimen consisting of cyclophosphamide/doxorubicin/methotrexate/procarbazine (CAMP). Among 486 patients, responses were seen in 31% with MVP, 25% with vindesine/cisplatin, 20% with etoposide/cisplatin, and 17% with CAMP. Survival was poorest with MVP (22 weeks), and only 26.6 weeks in the best group. Administration of MVP every 3 weeks to 121 patients resulted in 9 cases of serious pulmonary toxicity. In addition to demonstrating that no 'best' therapy existed for these patients, the study concluded that patients with an ECOG performance status of 2 are predisposed to excessive toxicity and poor survival (median, 10.4 weeks) and, therefore, should not be included in similar clinical trials.

The Indiana University study of 124 patients with unresectable NSCLC supported this conclusion [8]. Patients were randomized to receive vindesine alone, vindesine/cisplatin (120 mg/m^2), or vindesine/cisplatin (60 mg/m^2)/mitomycin (12 mg/m^2). The majority of patients in all

Table 3. Neoadjuvant therapy in patients with stage III NSCLC

Investigator	Ref.	Regimen	Patients n	Response %	Resected %	Median survival months
Gralla et al.	15	MVP	58	74	57	19
Henriquez et al.	16	MVP	53	68	49	10+
Burkes et al.	17	MVP	35	68.6	48.6	–
Elias et al.	18	CAP + RT	32	43 (to CAP)	65.6	31
Bitran et al.	19	Vindesine/cisplatin/etoposide	20	70	15	9
Sridhar et al.	20	Cisplatin/5-FU/etoposide + RT	21	68	73	12+

RT = Radiation therapy.

three treatment arms had a Karnofsky performance status of less than 80. No significant differences in survival, response rate, or response duration were noted. Among 41 patients treated with MVP, there were 4 toxic deaths, 2 due to pulmonary fibrosis and 2 to sepsis. Considerable hematologic toxicity was also observed in these patients.

In an attempt to assess the value of combination chemotherapy as compared with a 'minimal' treatment arm, the Southeastern Cancer Study Group randomized 453 patients to receive mitomycin (20 mg/m^2 on day 1, then 15 mg/m^2 every 6 weeks)/vindesine (3 mg/m^2/week × 5, then every 2 weeks), vindesine/cisplatin (120 mg/m^2), or lower doses of vindesine alone (the minimal treatment, or control, arm) [9]. All patients had advanced NSCLC unsuitable for resection or curative irradiation. In the 222 patients whose Karnofsky performance status was greater than 80, responses to chemotherapy were seen in 34% with mitomycin/vindesine and 22% with vindesine/cisplatin. No responses to single-agent vindesine were noted. Even in this group of good patients median survival was unaffected by treatment (23.5, 27.5, and 25.4 weeks for the mitomycin/vindesine, vindesine/cisplatin, and single-agent vindesine arms, respectively). The investigators concluded that, while individual patients may benefit from currently available combination chemotherapy, it does not meaningfully improve the survival of patients with advanced NSCLC.

These results conflict with those reported recently in a smaller randomized trial by the National Cancer Institute of Canada [14]. There patients treated with vindesine/cisplatin and CAP combinations were compared to a 'best supportive care' group that could receive palliative radiotherapy, antibiotics, and steroids. Virtually all patients had stage IV disease. Surprisingly, despite responses rates of only 25.3% for vindesine/cisplatin- and 15.3% for CAP-treated patients, a significant improvement in median survival was observed in the vindesine/cisplatin arm (32.6 weeks for vindesine/cisplatin vs. 24.7 weeks for CAP vs. 17 weeks for BSC; $p = 0.01$ for vindesine/cisplatin vs. BSC). While many studies have demonstrated that patients responding to chemotherapy show improvement in survival, this study further suggests that patients whose disease is only stabilized by chemotherapy may also obtain a survival benefit.

Mitomycin in Combined Modality Therapy

During the past 5 years several studies have investigated the use of combined modality treatment in patients with stage IIIA NSCLC [15–21]. Chemotherapy has been given simultaneously with radiation therapy or prior to either radiation or surgery. This neoadjuvant approach has yielded response rates higher than those previously reported in patients with advanced disease (table 3) [15–20]. The percent of patients undergoing surgical resection has been high in these studies, and it appears that chemotherapy can successfully downstage previously inoperable patients. Perhaps more important is the observation that as many as 15–30% of resected surgical specimens show no evidence of cancer [15, 16]. Follow-up of these complete responders has confirmed that their survival time is significantly longer than that for patients who have some residual tumor [21].

While studies in advanced NSCLC have suggested little survival benefit with MVP or any other drug combination, a review of the literature suggests that MVP combinations are associated with higher response rates than are other available regimens (table 4) [22], making MVP highly suitable for use in neoadjuvant therapy. This cer-

Table 4. Cisplatin combination chemotherapy in patients with metastatic NSCLC

Regimen	Patients n	Studies n	Response %
CAP	432	5	29
Vinca alkaloid/cisplatin	426	9	35
MVP	362	7	49
Etoposide/cisplatin	384	5	29

Adapted from Gralla [22].

Table 5. Comparative dose intensities for MVP regimens

Investigator	Dose intensity, mg/m²/week			Patients n	Response %
	mitomycin	vinca alkaloid	cisplatin		
Gralla et al., 1986	2	2.25	30	52[a]	54
ECOG, 1989	3.3	2	13	176[a]	20
Martini et al., 1987	2	2.25	30	58[b]	69
Burkes et al., 1988	2	2.25	30	23[b]	87
Wagner et al., 1985	3.3	2	13	42[b]	48

Patients had either stage IV[a] or III[b] NSCLC. Adapted from Bonomi et al. [23].

tainly represents an exciting new direction in the treatment of NSCLC for which randomized clinical trials are now required.

Conclusions

Mitomycin is one of the most active single agents available for the treatment of NSCLC. Studies have confirmed that combining this drug with vinca alkaloids and cisplatin (MVP) can achieve responses rates of greater than 50% in selected patients with good performance status. A wide range of results have been reported in numerous clinical trials of MVP. This may reflect differences among patient populations enrolled in these trials, but also reflects differences in the dose intensity of the agents used. Pharmacologic studies in animals have not suggested a steep dose-response curve with mitomycin [R.T. Dorr, PhD, personal commun., 1987]. Experience in our practice indicates that a reduction in dose from 10 to 7 or 8 mg/m² does not bring about a loss of efficacy and results in fewer hematologic and other toxicities. Additionally, we have noted that even lower doses of mitomycin (3–5 mg/m²) can induce and maintain remissions in other solid tumors (e.g., breast and cervical cancer). A comparative analysis of results reported using MVP regimens in NSCLC suggests that high response rates are associated with greater dose-intensive use of cisplatin and lesser dose-intensive use of mitomycin (table 5) [23]. This approach should be used in future clinical trials incorporating these drugs.

The most promising use of mitomycin combination chemotherapy is as part of a multidisciplinary approach to the treatment of stage IIIA NSCLC. The high response rates and complete remissions observed with short courses of MVP in several neoadjuvant trials have encouraged oncologists to adopt this approach in community practice. It is important that the validity of this approach be better defined with randomized clinical trials. Studies of adjuvant chemotherapy using short courses of MVP following surgical excision should also be undertaken. The high relapse rate in all but the earliest stages of NSCLC warrants such studies.

The role of the MVP regimen in patients with advanced NSCLC is unclear. Responding patients generally have

Table 6. Mitomycin regimens without platinum in advanced NSCLC

Investigator	Ref.	Regimen (mitomycin +)	Patients n	Response %	Median survival months
Bianco et al.	24	Vindesine/etoposide	40	40	6
Leudke et al.	9, 25	Vindesine	256	27.7	5
Miller et al.	27	5-FU/vincristine	56	41	5.5
Butler and Rosi et al.	28, 29	5-FU/doxorubicin	55	34.5	–
Kris et al.	26	EDAM/vinblastine	30	60	–

EDAM = 10-Ethyl-10-deazaaminopterin.

improvement in both performance status and survival, but responses are frequently short-lived, and the toxicity of high-dose cisplatin can be prohibitive for some patients. Physicians should discourage patients with poor performance status from receiving this therapy: they seldom derive a worthwhile benefit and are more likely to experience significant toxicity from treatment. Other mitomycin regimens without cisplatin have been studied and might be more appropriate in such patients desiring therapy (table 6) [10, 24–29]. Clearly, our focus must be on the discovery of new agents with greater activity and on approaches toward reducing the toxicity of available agents for patients with NSCLC.

References

1 Kris M, Cohen E, Gralla R: An analysis of 134 phase II trials in non-small cell lung cancer (NSCLC) (abstract). Proc IVth World Conf Lung Cancer, Toronto, 1985, p 133.

2 Bonomi P: Carboplatin in non-small cell lung cancer: Review of the Eastern Cooperative Oncology Group Trial and comparison with other carboplatin trials. Semin Oncol 1991; 18(suppl 2):2–7.

3 Bakowski MT, Creech JC: Chemotherapy of non-small cell lung cancer: A reappraisal and look to the future. Cancer Treat Rev 1983;10: 159–172.

4 Eagan RT, Ingle JN, Frytak S, et al: Platinum-based polychemotherapy versus dianhydrogalactitol in advanced non-small cell lung cancer. Cancer Treat Rep 1977;61:1339–1345.

5 Gralla R, Casper E, Kelson D, et al: Cisplatin and vindesine combination chemotherapy for advanced carcinoma of the lung: A randomized trial investigating two dosage schedules. Ann Intern Med 1981;95:414–420.

6 Gralla RJ, Kris MG, Burke MT, et al: The influence of the addition of mitomycin (M) to vindesine (V) plus cisplatin (P) in a random-assignment trial in 120 patients with non-small lung cancer (NSCLC) (abstract). Proc Am Soc Clin Oncol 1982;5:182.

7 Ruckdeschel JC, Finkelstein DM, Ettinger DS, et al: A randomized trial of the four most active regimens for metastatic non-small cell lung cancer. J Clin Oncol 1986;4:14–22.

8 Einhorn LH, Loehrer P, Williams SD, et al: Random prospective study of vindesine versus vindesine plus high-dose cisplatin versus vindesine plus cisplatin plus mitomycin-C in advanced non-small cell lung cancer. J Clin Oncol 1986;4:1037–1043.

9 Leudke DW, Einhorn L, Omura GA, et al: Randomized comparison of two combination regimens versus minimal chemotherapy in non-small cell lung cancer: A Southeastern Cancer Study Group trial. J Clin Oncol 1990; 8:886–891.

10 Hansen HH: Advanced non-small cell lung cancer: To treat or not to treat? J Clin Oncol 1987;5:1711–1712.

11 Folman RS, Rosman M: The role of chemotherapy in non-small cell lung cancer: The community perspective. Semin Oncol 1988; 15(suppl 4):16–21.

12 Gralla RJ, Kris MG, Potanovich LM, et al: Enhancing the safety and efficacy of the MVP regimen (mitomycin + vinblastine + cisplatin) in 100 patients with inoperable non-small cell lung cancer (abstract). Proc Am Soc Clin Oncol 1989;8:227.

13 Veeder M, Jett J, Therneau T: Phase III trial of mitomycin-C, velban, cisplatin (MVP) versus mitomycin-C alone (M) for metastatic squamous cell lung cancer (SqC) (abstract). Proc Am Soc Clin Oncol 1990;9:224.

14 Rapp E, Pater JL, Willan A, et al: Chemotherapy can prolong survival in patients with non-small cell lung cancer: Report of a Canadian multicenter randomized trial. J Clin Oncol 1988;6:633–641.

15 Gralla RJ, Kris MG, Martini N, et al: A neoadjuvant trial in stage IIIA non-small cell lung cancer in patients with clinically apparent mediastinal node involvement with MVP chemotherapy (mitomycin + vinca alkaloid + cisplatin) (abstract). Lung Cancer 1988;4(suppl): A161.

16 Henriquez I, Muñoz-Galindo L, Rebollo JM, et al: Neoadjuvant chemotherapy (NAC) with cisplatin (CDDP), mitomycin-C (MMC) and vindesine (VDS) in locally advanced non-small cell lung cancer (NSCLC) (abstract). Proc Am Soc Clin Oncol 1990;9:227.

17 Burkes R, Ginsberg R, Shepherd M, et al: Neo-adjuvant trial with MVP (Mitomycin-C + vindesine + cisplatin) chemotherapy for stage III (T1–3, N2, M0) unresectable non-small cell lung cancer (NSCLC) (abstract). Proc Am Soc Clin Oncol 1989;8:221.

18 Elias AD, Skarin AT, Socinski MA, et al: Neoadjuvant therapy for stage IIIA non-small cell lung cancer (NSCLC) (abstract). Proc Am Soc Clin Oncol 1989;8:241.

19 Bitran JD, Golumb HM, Hoffman PC, et al: Protochemotherapy in non-small cell lung carcinoma. An attempt to increase surgical resectability and survival. A preliminary report. Cancer 1986;57:44–53.
20 Sridhar KS, Thurer R, Kim Y, et al: Multimodality treatment of non-small cell lung cancer: Response to cisplatin, VP-16, and 5-FU chemotherapy and to surgery and radiation therapy. J Surg Oncol 1988;38:193–215.
21 Bonomi P, Gale M, Taylor SG IV, et al: Prognostic significance of histologic complete remission in neoadjuvant trials in stage 3 non-small cell lung cancer (NSCLC) (abstract). Proc Am Soc Clin Oncol 1990;9:230.
22 Gralla RJ: Issues and agents in the chemotherapy of non-small cell lung cancer. Mediguide Oncol 1985;5:1–5.
23 Bonomi PD, Finkelstein DM, Ruckdeschel JC, et al: Combination chemotherapy versus single agents followed by combination chemotherapy in stage IV non-small cell lung cancer: A study of the Eastern Cooperative Oncology Group. J Clin Oncol 1989;7:1602–1613.
24 Bianco AR, Gridelli C, Pepe R, et al: Phase II study of mitomycin-C, etoposide and vindesine in stage IV non-small cell lung cancer (NSCLC) (abstract). Proc Am Soc Clin Oncol 1990;9:233.
25 Leudke DW, Leudke SL, Martelo O, et al: Vindesine and mitomycin in the treatment of advanced non-small cell lung cancer: A Southeastern Cancer Study Group trial. Cancer Treat Rep 1986;70:651–653.
26 Kris MG, Gralla RJ, Potanovich LM, et al: Incorporating 10-ethyl-10-deazaaminopterin (EDAM) into combination therapy with mitomycin (M) and vinblastine (V) for patients (Pts) with advanced non-small cell lung cancer (NSCLC) (abstract). Proc Am Soc Clin Oncol 1989;8:227.
27 Miller TP, McMahan LJ, Livingston RB: Extensive adenocarcinoma and large cell undifferentiated carcinoma of the lung treated with 5-FU, vincristine and mitomycin-C (FOMi). Cancer Treat Rep 1980;64:1241–1245.
28 Butler TP, Macdonald JS, Smith FP, et al: 5-fluorouracil, Adriamycin, and mitomycin-C (FAM) chemotherapy for adenocarcinoma of the lung. Cancer 1979;43:1183–1188.
29 Rosi DR, Nogeire C, Brown B, et al: 5-Fluorouracil, Adriamycin, and mitomycin-C (Hi-FAM) chemotherapy for adenocarcinoma of the lung. Cancer 1981;48:21–25.

Oncology 1993;50(suppl 1):31–34

Michael H. Cullen

Queen Elizabeth Hospital
Birmingham, UK

Mitomycin, Ifosfamide, and Cisplatin in Non-Small Cell Lung Cancer

Key Words
Chemotherapy
Non-small cell lung cancer

Abstract
Mitomycin, ifosfamide, and cisplatin have demonstrated the best single-agent activity thus far in patients with non-small cell lung cancer (NSCLC), the most common malignant disease in the western world. For this reason, we initiated a phase II study, giving these three agents in combination (designated MIC) to 74 patients with inoperable NSCLC. Sixty-six patients were evaluable for response, of whom 30 (45%) demonstrated a partial response and 7 (11%) a complete response. These results, along with those obtained in two other phase II trials of MIC in NSCLC, prompted us to begin a large-scale, multicenter, phase III study of MIC in patients with inoperable limited-stage NSCLC. In this ongoing study, patients have been randomized to receive treatment with MIC and radiotherapy or radiotherapy alone. We hope to resolve the issue of whether a survival advantage is conferred on NSCLC patients treated with radiotherapy in combination with this promising chemotherapeutic regimen.

Non-small cell lung cancer (NSCLC) is the most common malignant disease in the western world and among the most chemoresistant. In tests of single-agent therapy in large patient cohorts, only 5 drugs – ifosfamide, mitomycin, cisplatin, vinblastine, and vindesine – have produced overall responses in 15% or more of cases [1]. The 3 most active agents, mitomycin, ifosfamide, and cisplatin, have been associated with response rates of 20, 26, and 20%, respectively (table 1) [2, 3]. We combined ifosfamide with mitomycin in a recent phase II study of patients with NSCLC [4]. Thirty patients were assessable for response to chemotherapy; 8 achieved partial remission (PR) and 5 complete remission (CR), for an overall response rate of 43%. Cisplatin and ifosfamide have demonstrated synergism in experimental models. Although both agents are associated with severe nausea and vomiting, a trial of antiemetic therapy in our unit [5] suggested that combining high-dose metoclopramide infusion, lorazepam, and dexamethasone would allow delivery of these drugs with acceptable subjective toxicity.

Patients and Methods

In January 1986 we began a phase II study of mitomycin/ifosfamide/cisplatin (MIC) in patients with inoperable NSCLC, the results of which have been previously reported [6]. In addition to assessing objective response, toxicity, and survival, we systematically monitored patients' performance status (PS) and body weight. Previously untreated ambulatory patients aged up to 70 years with inoperable, histologically confirmed, measurable or evaluable NSCLC were eligible. The vast majority of cases had squamous histology.

Michael H. Cullen, MD
Queen Elizabeth Hospital
Edgbaston
Birmingham B15 2TH (UK)

0030–2414/93/0507–0031
$2.75/0

The treatment schedule consisted of mitomycin 6 mg/m^2 by intravenous bolus infusion, ifosfamide 3 g/m^2 by i.v. infusion over 3 h, and cisplatin 50 mg/m^2 by i.v. infusion over 1 h. The complete schedule is given in table 2. Courses were repeated every 21 days. Responding patients who had not experienced unacceptable toxicity received a maximum of four courses. Those who failed to show objective and/or symptomatic improvement discontinued chemotherapy at any stage and were treated with radiotherapy. Responding patients with localized tumors received radiotherapy after chemotherapy. Patients were fully reassessed after a maximum of four chemotherapy courses. Response was assessed clinically and with chest X-ray in all cases, using World Health Organization (WHO) criteria. Body weight and WHO performance status were assessed before and 3 weeks after chemotherapy.

Results

Seventy-four patients entered this study; 66 were evaluable for response. Thirty patients (45%) achieved PR and 7 (11%) achieved CR as assessed radiologically. The overall response rate was thus 56% (95% confidence interval, CI, 44–68%). Twenty-nine of 43 patients with limited disease (67%; 95% CI, 53–81%) and 8 of 23 with extensive disease (35%; 95% CI, 15–55%) responded to

Table 1. Response rates in NSCLC (drugs studied in >100 patients)

Drug	Trials n	Responders, n/ evaluable, n	Mean response rate	
			%	range
Ifosfamide	4	62/237	26	7–32
Cisplatin	5	28/140	20	6–32
Mitomycin	4	23/115	20	9–40
Vindesine	9	49/288	17	6–31
Doxorubicin	5	34/261	13	6–38
Dibromodulcitol	1	15/115	13	–
Baker's antifol (Triazinate)	3	14/119	12	5–15
Etoposide	4	21/195	11	3–21
Hexamethylmelamine	3	18/166	11	0–17
Methotrexate	6	25/247	10	0–26
Cyclophosphamide	5	3/369	8	4–42
Mechlorethamine	1	9/109	8	–
Carboplatin	12	32/439	7	0–9
Lomustine	4	12/161	7	2–28
Amsacrine	3	6/143	4	0–7
Chlorozotocin	3	3/128	2	0–7

Adapted from Bakowski and Creach [2] and Bunn [3].

Table 2. MIC chemotherapy regimen (Queen Elizabeth Hospital)

Time, h	Regimen	
0	Metoclopramide 1 mg/kg i.v. in 100 ml 0.9% saline over 30 min	
0.5	Dexamethasone 8 mg in 50 ml 0.9% saline i.v. over 15 min Lorazepam 2 mg/m^2 in 50 ml 0.9% saline over 15 min	
1.0	Metoclopramide 9 mg/kg i.v. given over 24 h by infusion pump Mitomycin 6 mg/m^2 i.v. bolus infusion	
	Ifosfamide 3 g/m^2 + mesna 1.0 g/m^2 in 1 liter 0.9% saline over 3 h	
4.0	Furosemide 40 mg p.o. Dexamethasone 4 mg in 50 ml 0.9% saline short infusion, then 1 liter 0.9% saline + 20 mmol potassium chloride	over 3 h
7.0	Mesna 500 mg/m^2 in 50 ml 0.9% saline short infusion, then cisplatin 50 mg/m^2 i.v. in 250 ml 0.9% saline	over 1 h
8.0	Dexamethasone 4 mg in 50 ml 0.9% saline short infusion, then mesna 500 mg/m^2 in 50 ml then 1 liter 0.9% saline + 20 mmol potassium chloride	over 6 h
12.0 16.0 20.0 24.0	Dexamethasone 4 mg in 50 ml 0.9% saline over 10 min	

Adapted from Cullen et al. [6].

treatment. The duration of response (to chemotherapy plus radiotherapy where given), measured from the start of treatment, was 8.75 months and median overall survival was 9.2 months. Responders survived a median of 12 months and nonresponders 5 months.

Toxicity was generally mild and consisted primarily of nausea and vomiting. Six of 67 evaluable patients experienced severe or prolonged (>48 h) nausea and vomiting after one or more courses of MIC, and 1 patient declined further therapy. Ten patients had no nausea or vomiting. For the remainder, it was mild and short-lived. Hematologic toxicity was monitored prior to each of 213 courses and during the nadir phase (days 8–16) in 130 courses. Leukopenia (WBC $<3.0 \times 10^9$/l) and/or thrombocytopenia (platelet count $<100 \times 10^9$/l) occurred in the nadir period during administration of 48% of courses, but in only 8% of patients did this persist to day 21 and delay further treatment. Two patients with leukopenia-related infections required hospitalization and 1 patient with treatment-related infection died during the leukopenic phase. Anemia (hemoglobin <10 g/dl) was present following administration of 28% of total courses, and raised serum creatinine levels (>125 μmol/l) were noted after 5%. All patients receiving two or more courses experienced alopecia.

Thirty-one responders and 28 nonresponders were evaluable for PS assessments. Fifteen responders improved their PS and only 1 responder deteriorated (fig. 1). Twenty-one of the 28 evaluable nonresponders had no change in PS, 3 increased, and 4 decreased. The difference in PS scores between responders and nonresponders was highly significant ($p = 0.002$). There was no difference in body weight between responders and nonresponders before treatment. Thirty evaluable responders experienced a mean weight gain of 2.9% with treatment, whereas 24 evaluable nonresponders had a mean weight loss of 3.8% (fig. 2). The difference in this change was also highly significant ($p = 0.0013$). The overall response rate of 56% (11% CR) suggests that the MIC combination is among the most active yet reported in the treatment of NSCLC.

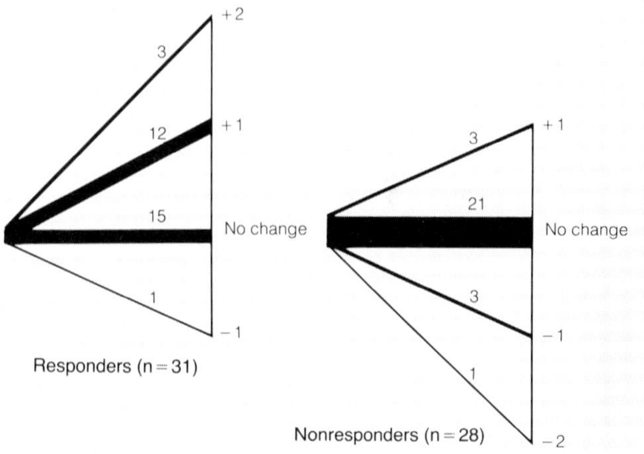

Fig. 1. Change in WHO PS score from start of treatment to 3 weeks after final course of MIC in 31 responders and 28 nonresponders. The difference in PS scores between responders and nonresponders was highly significant ($p = 0.002$).

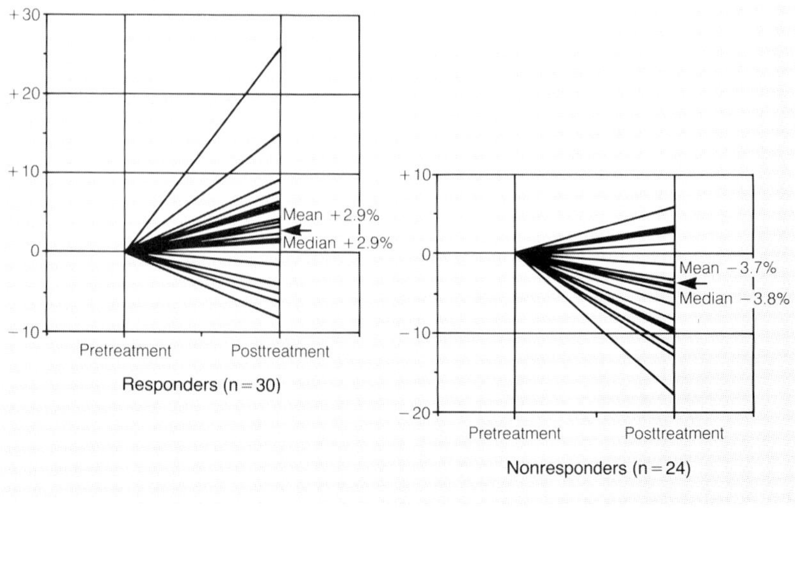

Fig. 2. Percent change in body weight from start of treatment to 3 weeks after final course of MIC in 30 responders and 24 nonresponders. The difference in weight change between responders and nonresponders was highly significant ($p = 0.0013$). Adapted from Cullen et al. [6].

Other Phase II Studies with MIC

Two other studies have tested MIC in patients with inoperable NSCLC. Giron et al. [7] reported results obtained in 32 cases, and Miles et al. [8] published an abstract describing a study of 45 cases. Thus, data exist for a total of 143 patients treated at three centers (Birmingham, Madrid [7], and London [8]). The total CR rate to date is 13% (18 of 143) and the PR rate is 41% (59 of 143), for an overall response rate of 54% (table 3) [6–8]. The London group used doses and schedules identical to those used in our study, whereas the Madrid group used higher doses of ifosfamide and cisplatin (and achieved higher response rates).

MIC in Phase III Studies

The results of the phase II data presented here prompted the establishment of a major collaborative randomized trial of MIC in patients with inoperable NSCLC. A number of centers in the United Kingdom are taking part in this trial, which began in 1988. The main participants are our group in Birmingham and the London-based lung cancer trials group. As of February 15, 1990, 220 patients have been accrued. Patients must have inoperable, previously untreated NSCLC categorized as limited-stage disease, for which the standard treatment in the United Kingdom would usually be radical radiotherapy. In this trial, patients are randomly assigned to treatment with MIC (maximum four courses) followed by radiotherapy or radiotherapy alone.

Table 3. Published response data on MIC in NSCLC

Investigator	Ref.	Evaluable patients n	CR %	PR %	OR %
Giron et al.	7	32	22	47	69
Cullen et al.	6	66	11	45	56
Miles et al.	8	45	9	31	40
Total		143	13	41	54

OR = Overall response.

Conclusion

The data on overall response and changes in body weight and PS reported in our phase II study imply not only that MIC is active and worthwhile for responders, but also that nonresponders do not experience any severe adverse reactions from exposure to chemotherapy. We believe this is because the doses of MIC were not excessive, the antiemetic schedule was intensive and largely effective, and nonresponders were promptly withdrawn from further treatment. The question of whether a survival advantage is conferred on patients with NSCLC treated with MIC and radiotherapy will be answered only when results from the large-scale randomized phase III trial are available.

References

1 Kris M, Cohen E, Gralla R: An analysis of 134 phase II trials in non-small cell lung cancer (NSCLC) (abstract). Proc 4th World Conf Lung Cancer. Toronto, August 25–30, 1985, vol 4, p 39.

2 Bakowski MT, Creach JC: Chemotherapy of non-small cell cancer: A reappraisal and a look to the future. Cancer Treat Rev 1983;10:159–172.

3 Bunn PA: Review of therapeutic trials of carboplatin in lung cancer. Semin Oncol 1990; 16(suppl 5):27–33.

4 Chetiyawardana AD, Cullen MH, Joshi RC, et al: Ifosfamide, mitomycin and radiotherapy in non-small cell lung cancer (NSCLC). Cancer Chemother Pharmacol 1989;24:102–104.

5 O'Brien MER, Cullen MH, Woodroffe CM, et al: The role of metoclopramide in acute and delayed chemotherapy induced emesis: A randomised double blind trial. Br J Cancer 1989; 60:759–763.

6 Cullen MH, Joshi R, Chetiyawardana AD, et al: Mitomycin, ifosfamide and cisplatin in non-small cell lung cancer: Treatment good enough to compare. Br J Cancer 1988;58:359–361.

7 Giron CG, Ordonez A, Jalon JI, et al: Combination chemotherapy with ifosfamide, mitomycin and cisplatin in advanced non-small cell lung cancer. Cancer Treat Rep 1987;71:851–853.

8 Miles DW, Earl HM, Drake J, et al: Combination chemotherapy with mitomycin, ifosfamide and cisplatin in non-small cell lung cancer (abstract). Br J Cancer 1990;61:183.

Oncology 1993;50(suppl 1):35–52

Robert C. Spain

Division of Oncology, St. Luke's Hospital, Cleveland, OH, USA

The Case for Mitomycin in Non-Small Cell Lung Cancer

Key Words

Mitomycin
Non-small cell lung cancer
Mitomycin in combined-modality therapy
Mitomycin-associated toxicity
Avoidance of mitomycin-associated toxicity

Abstract

The activity of mitomycin in non-small cell lung cancer (NSCLC) has been well documented in both single-institution pilot and multi-institution randomized trials. Despite the inclusion of patients ineligible for current trials of newer single agents due to poor performance status, prior irradiation to indicator lesions, or prior chemotherapy, mitomycin emerges from such prior studies as the most consistently active single agent currently available for NSCLC. While randomized trials in stage IV disease demonstrate an improved response rate with mitomycin and cisplatin in comparison with cisplatin alone ($p = 0.03$), and with mitomycin, vindesine, and cisplatin in comparison with vindesine and cisplatin alone ($p = 0.003$), the potential with mitomycin is most apparent with weekly bolus or infused vindesine/vinblastine, and higher-dose cisplatin (MVP) in neoadjuvant approaches to stage III disease. Indeed, four trials of neoadjuvant MVP in predominantly stage IIIA (bulky N2) disease produced a consistent 19-month median and 26–33% 3-year survival, which is to be compared with 8 months and 6%, respectively, with traditional thoracic irradiation alone. Nonetheless, prior use of mitomycin without guidelines for cumulative dose, schedule, or guidelines for use in combined-modality therapy has produced widespread frustration stemming not only from frequent antineoplastic effect, but also from frequent toxicity. The several related syndromes of mitomycin-associated thrombotic microangiopathy, ranging from hemolytic-uremic syndrome to pulmonary injury, appear avoidable through limiting the cumulative mitomycin dose to a maximum of 30 mg/m^2; scheduling mitomycin at not less than 4- to 6-week intervals; perioperative use of corticosteroids and low inspired oxygen; and close patient follow-up. While dexamethasone preceding mitomycin reduces the frequency and severity of mitomycin-associated lung injury ($p = 0.0005$), dexamethasone premedication also reduces the response rate of MVP in NSCLC ($p < 0.025$).

Significant advances have been achieved over the past decade in chemotherapy for non-small cell lung cancer (NSCLC). Improvements include the identification of chemotherapeutic agents with appreciable single-agent activity [1], identification of chemotherapeutic combinations that not only produce objective regression of measurable NSCLC [2, 3] but also improve survival in comparison with supportive care alone [4], demonstration of the feasibility of chemotherapy in combined-modality or neoadjuvant therapy [5, 6] and recognition of individual

Robert C. Spain, MD
Division of Oncology
St. Luke's Hospital
1311 Shaker Boulevard
Cleveland, OH 44104 (USA)

0030–2414/93/0507–0035
$2.75/0

patient characteristics – notably lower stage of disease – predictive of greater sensitivity to chemotherapy and potential for prolonged survival [7–11].

Despite these improvements, chemotherapy for NSCLC remains challenging. Although active agents are available, the administration of those agents, and their optimal doses, requires attention to detail. Illustrative of this is the fact that mitomycin, in single-agent studies, is the most consistently active antineoplastic drug currently available for the treatment of NSCLC [12–16]. High-dose cisplatin-'based' combination chemotherapy is considered superior to regimens previously available [2, 8, 17, 18]. Furthermore, four studies from three nations involving a total of 210 patients strongly suggest a meaningful survival advantage with neoadjuvant mitomycin, weekly or infused vinblastine/vindesine, and higher-dose cisplatin (MVP) for locoregionally advanced, stage III NSCLC [19–23]. Nonetheless, the literature is replete with the unfortunate consequences of incorrectly administered mitomycin and cisplatin, either as single agents or in combination. Furthermore, numerous reports have detailed the development of sepsis and/or respiratory insufficiency following MVP and subsequent radiation therapy or surgical resection. While guidelines for the reliable use of optimal doses of cisplatin are readily available [24–26], there are no clear instructions for the successful use of mitomycin, nor for the use of MVP in combined-modality therapy.

The chronology of mitomycin-containing combination chemotherapy has been confusing. In early protocols the mitomycin dosing interval was often short, the drug being administered too frequently, and to a large cumulative dose. As a result, response rates were moderate but toxicity occurred frequently, and there was only a minimal effect on survival. Subsequent attempts to avoid toxicity by increasing the mitomycin dosing interval led to reliance on less-active chemotherapeutic agents, which in turn produced low response rates and minimal effect on survival.

From this aggregate experience mitomycin has emerged as a paradox: An agent with intriguing chemotherapeutic activity in a traditionally chemotherapy-refractory disease but as well an agent associated with a significant incidence of toxicity. Perhaps most frustrating, toxicity appears to develop most commonly among patients responding well to mitomycin-containing therapy. For these several reasons, the role of mitomycin in NSCLC, particularly combined-modality management of stage III NSCLC, remains the subject of considerable controversy in both academic centers and community practice.

This report reviews the activity of single-agent mitomycin in NSCLC, the effect of adding mitomycin to vinca alkaloids or cisplatin, the effect of adding mitomycin to vinca alkaloids *and* cisplatin, the rationale for neoadjuvant management of stage III NSCLC, and the cumulative international experience with neoadjuvant mitomycin/cisplatin/vinblastine for locoregionally advanced stage III NSCLC. In addition, practical suggestions are offered for realizing the advantages of mitomycin and avoiding the complications.

Single-Agent Mitomycin

Published studies of single-agent mitomycin administered by intermittent bolus are listed in table 1. The frequently cited experience of Whittington and Close [27] with daily, chronic low-dose mitomycin has been excluded as an inferior regimen that is no longer applicable. Three of the five trials in table 1 are prospective randomized trials conducted in either single-institution [15] or multi-institution national cooperative group [13, 16] settings. In all three trials, stringent criteria of response were applied. Included within the five series are patients with prior chemotherapy, prior radiation therapy to indicator lesions, and patients with suboptimal Eastern Cooperative Oncology Group (ECOG) performance status of 2 and 3, criteria that would render patients ineligible for current single-agent studies. Patients who received prior chemotherapy were enrolled in at least two of the series in table 1 [12, 14], patients with prior radiotherapy to indicator lesions were in two series [14, 15], and patients with prior radiotherapy were entered in all five series.

Despite the suboptimal features of the patient populations studied, several points can be drawn from the data in table 1. First, at the doses and schedules studied, mitomycin has reasonable and reproducible single-agent activity (19–36%). Considering other single agents, etoposide, for example, has demonstrated variable and frequently minimal activity at conventional doses and schedules [28]. In two studies, addition of etoposide to cisplatin or carboplatin did not result in meaningful improvement in activity over that achieved with either platinum analogue alone [29, 30]. Vinca alkaloids similarly have shown inconsistent (7–33%) response rates [31–33] and single-agent carboplatin has inconsistently produced responses (0–20%) in addition to having a variable influence on survival in stage III and IV disease [30, 34–37]. Ifosfamide [38, 39] and cisplatin [40–43] also have demonstrated variable activity as single agents. Thus, mitomycin emerges

Table 1. Single-agent mitomycin in NSCLC

Authors	Ref.	Patients n	Stage	ECOG performance status	Cell type	Dose (mg/m^2), schedule	Response %	Cycles to response	Duration of response/ survival, weeks
Samson et al.	12	35	'Incurable'	0–3	Large cell/ adenocarcinoma	20, q6wk	20	1	12/
ECOG	13	27	III 36% IV 64%	0–3	Squamous cell	20, q3wk	19		/12
Koons et al.	14	28	Recurrent 'inoperable'	1–3	Squamous cell	20, q4wk	36	1–2	14+/18+
Niell et al.	15	53	III 19% IV 81%	0–2	NSCLC	10, q4wk	19		16/23
NCCTG	16	64	III 13% IV 87%	0–3	Squamous cell	20, 15, q4wk	30		16/16
Total		207					51/207, 25%		

as the most consistently active chemotherapeutic agent currently available in single-agent studies of NSCLC.

Second, it is also clear from table 1 that mitomycin activity, if present, becomes evident quickly. Samson et al. [12] noted that all therapeutic responses were apparent within the initial course of single-agent mitomycin. Similarly, Koons et al. [14] observed some indication of tumor reduction with the initial mitomycin dose in 9 of 10 ultimate responders. They further observed that no patient whose disease was stable following 2 cycles of mitomycin subsequently established a clear response with a 3rd or further dose. This is consistent with the observation that any activity of combination mitomycin/cisplatin/vinca alkaloid for NSCLC becomes evident within the 1st or 2nd course and further supports observations by Walters et al. [44] and Creech et al. [45] who reported comparable rapid response to mitomycin by breast cancer patients. Thus, patients who are likely, or unlikely, to benefit from continued therapy with mitomycin can be identified early in their treatment.

While the activity of single-agent mitomycin listed in table 1 was obtained with doses of 10–20 mg/m^2, no data are available regarding activity with 6–8 mg/m^2, as is commonly used in combination chemotherapy. Numerous reports have suggested the squamous cell variety of NSCLC to be more responsive to mitomycin either as a single agent or in combination chemotherapy [3, 11, 14, 16, 46, 47]. Finally, although response and survival are brief in the available single-agent mitomycin studies, this is not too surprising in view of the inclusion of patients with suboptimal performance status and prior treatment.

Mitomycin and Vinca Alkaloids, Mitomycin and Cisplatin

Several groups have studied mitomycin in combination with vindesine or vinblastine (table 2) [48–54]. Although it is potentially hazardous to compare different series, the addition of vindesine or vinblastine to mitomycin appears to produce only a modest improvement in activity and survival compared with the effects of mitomycin alone. It should be kept in mind, however, that these studies included patients with suboptimal ECOG performance status 2 and 3 and, frequently, prior radiotherapy (not analyzed separately in four of the trials). The mitomycin/ vinca alkaloid combinations are generally well tolerated and thus can be readily administered to outpatients deemed unable to tolerate cisplatin.

The Southwest Oncology Group [42] randomized patients with stage IV disease to mitomycin and cisplatin versus cisplatin alone. While the mitomycin-cisplatin combination was clearly more active ($p = 0.03$), median survival was only minimally improved by the addition of mitomycin to cisplatin.

Table 2. Mitomycin and vinca alkaloids

Investigator	Ref.	Patients n	Stage	Patients %	ECOG performance status	Dose (mg/m^2), schedule	Response rate, %	Median survival weeks
SECSG	48	59	'Incurable'		–	Mitomycin 20,15, q6wk Vindesine 3 qwk × 6 then 3 q2wk	36	–
SECSG	49	122	III IV	43 57	0–2	Same as above	27	20.4
Kris et al.	50	Prior CT 29	III IV	7 93	1–2	Mitomycin 10, days 1, 21, 57 then q6wk × 2 then q8wk	Prior CT 17 (5/29)	21
		No prior CT 55	III IV	11 89	1–2	Vindesine 3, qwk × 5 then q2wk	No prior CT 36 (20/55)	27
SWOG	51	45	IV		0–3	Mitomycin 10, q3wk Vinblastine 1, q12h × 4 q3wk	24 and 24 'improved'	19
Shinkai et al.	52	No prior therapy 30	III IV	33 67	0–3	Mitomycin 8, qwk × 3 then q3wk Vindesine 3, qwk × 5 then q2wk	10	44
Sculier et al.	53	Prior RT/CT 16	III IV	31 69	0–2	Mitomycin 15, 10, q4wk	6 (1/16)	19
		No prior therapy 27	III IV	29 71	0–2	Vindesine 3, qwk × 3 then q2wk	33 (9/27)	22
Gatzemeier et al.	54	No prior therapy 66	IIIB IV	17 83	0–3	Mitomycin 10, day 1, q4wk Vindesine 3, day 1, 8 q4wk	23	23

CT = Chemotherapy, RT = radiotherapy. Values in parentheses = n patients/total.

Mitomycin/Cisplatin/Vinca Alkaloids (MVP)

The Memorial Sloan-Kettering group has addressed the question of whether mitomycin improves the activity of cisplatin and the vinca alkaloid vindesine in stage III and IV disease (table 3) [2, 3, 55]. In all three studies the same doses and schedules of vindesine and cisplatin were used regardless of the inclusion of mitomycin in the study regimen. In comparing sequential studies of the initial 2-drug and the subsequent 3-drug combination, and thereafter in a phase III trial prospectively randomizing patients to the 2-drug versus 3-drug combination, response rates were significantly improved with the addition of mitomycin. Median survival, however, was 46–52 weeks in both treatment groups.

Other attempts to measure the effect of adding mitomycin to cisplatin and vindesine or vinblastine have compared different doses and schedules of cisplatin and the vinca alkaloid in the 2-drug and 3-drug combinations. Determination of the impact of mitomycin is difficult under such variable conditions.

Widely varying results have been reported with MVP for advanced NSCLC. Clearly, there are major differences in the dose and schedule of mitomycin, cisplatin, and vindesine or vinblastine in the various regimens, each referred to as MVP. Furthermore, there are major differences in performance status, specific stage of disease, and prior treatment of the subjects studied. It is not surprising that different response rates, response durations, and survival times are observed when widely varying chemotherapy regimens are applied to different patient populations.

Table 3. Mitomycin plus cisplatin/vindesine for stage III and IV NSCLC[1]

Investigator	Ref.	Patients n	Dose, mg/m²	Schedule	Response, %
Sequential phase II trials					
Gralla et al.	2	40	Cisplatin 120 Vindesine 3	Days 1, 29, then q6wk qwk × 6, then q2wk	40
Kris et al.	3	87	Mitomycin 8 Cisplatin 120 Vindesine 3	Days 1, 29, 71 Days 1, 29, 71 qwk × 5, then q2wk	60
*Randomized trial**					
Gralla et al.	55	111	Cisplatin 120 Vindesine 3	Days 1, 29, then q6wk qwk × 5, then q2wk	27
				versus	
			Mitomycin 8 Cisplatin 120 Vindesine 3	Days 1, 29, 71 Days 1, 29, 71 qwk × 5, then q2wk	54

* p = 0.003.
[1] Memorial Sloan-Kettering Cancer Center.

Rationale for Neoadjuvant Therapy for Stage III NSCLC

Approximately 40% of NSCLC patients present with demonstrable disease 'limited' to one hemithorax but with mediastinal and/or supraclavicular lymphatic involvement and/or direct mediastinal extension of primary tumor, and thus disease too advanced for surgical resection [56, 57]. Limited yet inoperable NSCLC, including stage IIIA disease with ipsilateral mediastinal lymphatic involvement (N2) and stage IIIB with contralateral mediastinal and/or supraclavicular involvement (N3) [58], has traditionally been managed with thoracic irradiation alone, which although effective in palliation, has little impact on long-term survival [31, 59, 60]. Mediastinal lymphatic involvement is the most certain indication of occult systemic micrometastasis [61]. With locoregional management alone the relapse rate is high and patterns of recurrence are predominantly distant, outside the surgical field and/or radiotherapy portal [59–64]. Systemic micrometastases are a major component of stage III NSCLC, and successful management requires effective systemic as well as locoregional therapy.

Neoadjuvant therapy refers to initial systemic and subsequent locoregional management, with as little time between the two as is possible [65]. Induction chemotherapy and subsequent consolidation with radiotherapy or resection address distant micrometastatic and bulky intrathoracic disease as well as the problem of incomplete intrathoracic control with single-modality therapy. Although locoregionally advanced (stage III) and distant metastatic (stage IV) disease are often lumped together as inoperable and therefore poor-prognosis NSCLC, there is reason to consider stage III disease as clinically distinct with unique therapeutic opportunities. Patients with stage III disease, who frequently experience less pretreatment weight loss and have a better performance status, generally are able to tolerate and are more likely to respond to more intensive therapy. This partially explains the common observation that stage III disease is more responsive to chemotherapy. While responses with currently available chemotherapy tend to be relatively brief, neoadjuvant approaches apply a potentially non-cross-resistant second therapeutic modality to the complete extent of disease demonstrable at original diagnosis, and thus provide more durable disease control. It is in the setting of combined-modality therapy that significant impact can currently be made, including prolongation of survival.

While the theoretical advantages of neoadjuvant therapy are intuitive and clear, the practical application is frequently difficult in elderly, fragile patients often compromised in lung function. Neoadjuvant therapy includes at least two forms of treatment, each of which must achieve maximal antineoplastic effect. Of equal significance, each modality must be sufficiently tolerable to allow definitive application of the second form of treatment. Specifically, primary chemotherapy must not only eliminate distant micrometastases and reduce bulky intrathoracic NSCLC, a disease notoriously refractory to chemotherapy, but also must be tolerated well enough to allow subsequent radiotherapy or surgery with curative intent. Herein lies the frustrating enigma of mitomycin. Although recognized as an active chemotherapeutic agent for NSCLC, mitomycin is also associated with pulmonary toxicity. In the absence of measures to avoid lung injury, mitomycin may compromise the administration of the critical second half of neoadjuvant therapy – potentially curative surgical resection or radiotherapy.

Neoadjuvant MPV: The Penrose Experience

In 1981 studies of neoadjuvant approaches to NSCLC were begun in Colorado Springs, Colorado [22]. From 1981 to 1985, 31 patients with locoregionally advanced disease were evaluated by thoracic surgeons, found to be inoperable or unresectable, and enrolled in a study of neoadjuvant therapy with mitomycin, cisplatin, and vinblastine, originally described as MPV [22].

Patients were deemed inoperable/unresectable due to the following anatomic extent of disease: (1) 14 with bulky N2 disease evident on chest roentgenogram or at bronchoscopy [stage IIIA (bulky N2), 14/31 (45%)]; (2) 13 with direct extension of primary tumor into the mediastinum with involvement of great vessels (T4); 1 with contralateral mediastinal lymphadenopathy (N3): 1 with bilateral supraclavicular lymphadenopathy (N3); [stage IIIB, 15/31 (48%)]; and (3) 2 with biopsy-proven local metastasis to ipsilateral lung or rib, discontinuous from primary tumor ['local' stage IV, 2/31 (7%)]. Four of the 31 patients were enrolled after being found unresectable at thoracotomy.

This was not a highly selected series. In the group treated with primary MPV and subsequent radiotherapy, four patients had Karnofsky performance statuses of 50–60%, 7 individuals were between the ages of 70 and 77 years, and 6 had severe chronic obstructive pulmonary disease (COPD) (forced expiratory volume in 1 s/forced vital capacity [FEV_1/FVC] 35–54%).

The specific doses of individual MPV agents were tailored to patient age and performance score (table 4). Less ambulatory patients were given lower doses of mitomycin and cisplatin. Vinblastine, a cell-cycle-specific agent with a short half-life [66], was administered as a 1 mg/m^2 bolus followed by a 6- to 7-day continuous infusion via central venous catheter and portable pump, primarily to outpatients. The sequencing of chemotherapy with radiotherapy was not identical in all neoadjuvant patients. Early in the study, 4 patients received radiotherapy followed immediately by 3–4 courses of MPV, and 5 received radiotherapy concurrent with their initial 2 courses of MPV. However, the majority of patients in the neoadjuvant series received the now-standard primary MPV followed by radiotherapy or resection. For survival analysis, all 31 patients were combined.

Table 4. Mitomycin, cisplatin and continuous-infusion vinblastine: Dosage variation with age and ECOG performance status

Patient characteristics	Mitomycin day 1, mg/m^2	Cisplatin day 5, mg/m^2	Vinblastine day 5, mg/m^2
			Days 5–12
Age ≤58 years	10	110	1, bolus
Performance status 0, 1, 2			1, qd × 7
			Days 5–11
Age 59–69 years	9	100	1, bolus
Performance status 0, 1, 2			1, qd × 6
			Days 5–11
Age ≥70 years	8	90	1, bolus
Performance status 0, 1, 2, 3			1, qd × 6

Although prospective randomization between neoadjuvant therapy and conventional radiotherapy alone would perhaps be the optimal means of assessing the contribution of primary MPV, a phase III trial was not possible in the community hospital in which this study was conducted in the early and mid 1980s. In view of the many uncertainties surrounding primary chemotherapy for NSCLC even at present, random assignment to neoadjuvant therapy versus radiotherapy alone would have been inappropriate in 1981. However, from 1979 through 1985, 60 patients with limited-stage yet anatomically inoperable NSCLC with performance statuses ≥60% and no pleural effusion were referred to Penrose Hospital by their private physicians for treatment with definitive radiotherapy alone. These patients were treated by the same radiation therapists, in the same institution, on the same equipment and during the same period of time as 26 neoadjuvant protocol patients who received MPV and radiotherapy (see below). Patients from the group referred for radiotherapy alone were individually matched with neoadjuvant patients according to equal prognostic fac-

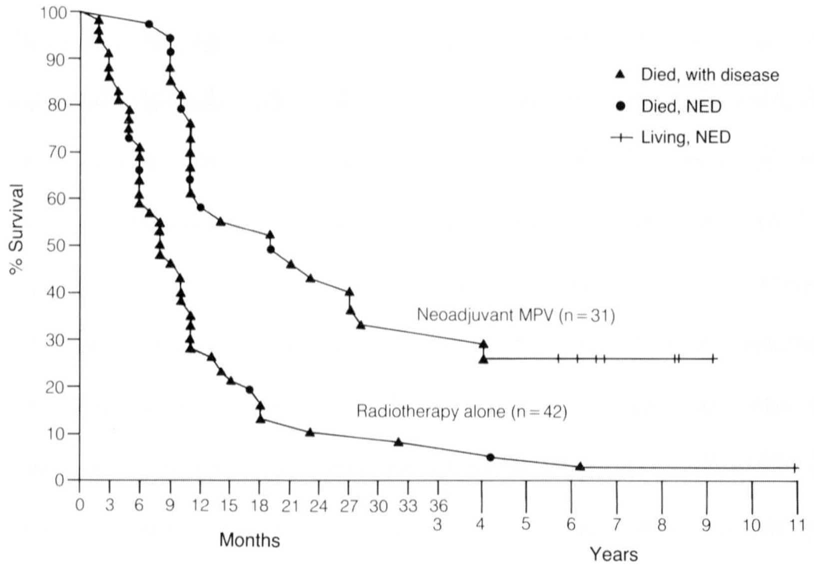

Fig. 1. Comparison of survival distribution with neoadjuvant MPV versus radiotherapy alone; $p < 0.001$. NED = No evidence of disease.

tors, including performance score, TNM extent of stage III NSCLC, weight loss prior to treatment, age, sex, and cell differentiation. In this manner, 42 radiotherapy-only patients were matched with 31 neoadjuvant patients with equal prognoses. All patients were followed for survival.

In both groups, radiotherapy consisted of 50–66 Gy conventional fractionation to areas of pulmonary involvement and 50 Gy to regional lymphatic drainage via four MEV linear accelerator or cobalt 60 teletherapy units. In neoadjuvant patients all radiation was administered to portals corresponding to prechemotherapy tumor dimensions.

Response to MPV

Of 22 subjects receiving primary MPV, a clinical complete response (CR) was obtained in 3 patients with squamous cell and 2 with large cell disease. Partial responses (PRs) were seen in 11 patients. Thus, a major response occurred in 16 of 22 (73%). No patient developed progressive disease prior to local consolidation.

In all responders, sensitivity to MPV was apparent within the first 2 courses and in the majority was evident within the 1st course. The maximum clinically apparent response occurred within 3 courses. In 10 patients a 4th course given prior to consolidation did not produce further clinically apparent tumor regression but was associated with lung injury following consolidation in 4 of the 10.

MPV and Resection

Surgical resection was not a primary objective of this study. Rather, the form of consolidation considered both tolerable and most likely to achieve local control in the individual patient was used. Five patients with a CR or PR to primary MPV underwent subsequent thoracotomy. Following MPV treatments, 2 patients who had been unresectable at thoracotomy prior to protocol entry were completely resected with a wedge resection and lobectomy. In 2 other patients definitive lobectomies were performed. The 5th patient became operable following MPV, but remained unresectable. Microscopic or macroscopic NSCLC was found in all 4 resected patients. Two of the 4 resected patients currently survive and remain active with no evidence of NSCLC at 80+ and 99+ months from initial MPV.

MPV and Thoracic Irradiation

Median survival in the 26 patients treated with radiotherapy rather than surgical resection is 19 months (range, 7–109), and 5 survive with no evidence of NSCLC 68, 73, 78, 99, and 109+ months from initial therapy.

Neoadjuvant Therapy versus Radiotherapy Alone

Median follow-up from initial therapy is currently more than 81 months in the entire neoadjuvant group and 101 months in the group treated with radiotherapy alone (fig. 1). Median survival of the 31 neoadjuvant-treated pa-

Table 5. Neoadjuvant MPV: the international experience

Investigator	Ref.	Patients n	Stage (%)*	Karnofsky performance status	Response rate, %	Consolidation		Median survival months	Three-year survival %	Six-year survival %
						Resected	%			
Pisters et al. Gralla	19 20	73	IIIA (100) 'clinical N2'	60–90	77	Surgery ±RT	60	19	26	–
Burkes et al.	21	39	IIIA (100) 'clinical N2'	Medically fit	64	Surgery	46	19	26	–
Spain (Penrose experience)	22	31	IIIA (45) 'bulky N2' IIIB (48) 'local IV' (7)	60–90	73	Surgery or RT	4/5	19	33	23
Henriquez et al.	23	71	IIIA (75) IIIB (25)	60–90	72	Surgery ±RT	52	>13	–	–

* Percent patients in parentheses.

tients is 19 months (range, 7–109). Three- and 6-year survivals are 33 and 23%, respectively, and the median duration of treatment-free survival is 13.5 months. Seven patients (23%) currently survive with no evidence of NSCLC 68–109 months from initial therapy. Seven patients died with no clinical evidence of NSCLC. Postmortem examination of 6 of these 7 patients revealed no evidence of NSCLC in 3 and only microscopic disease in 3.

In contrast, median survival with radiotherapy alone is 8 months, and 3- and 6-year survivals are 6 and 3%, respectively. One patient survives without evidence of disease at more than 131 months from initial radiotherapy. The difference in survival distributions with neoadjuvant management versus radiotherapy alone is statistically significant ($p < 0.0001$).

Myelosuppression due to MPV

Myelosuppression associated with MPV was cumulative and significant. Median absolute granulocyte nadirs following the 1st, 2nd, and 3rd courses were 803, 427, and 243×10^6/L, respectively. With 103 courses of MPV administered, 8 episodes of leukopenic fever developed in 6 patients. No septic deaths occurred in relation to MPV.

Neoadjuvant MVP: The International Experience

Among the four phase II series in table 5, which includes the study discussed above, there are several common features in the dosing and scheduling of MVP. Mitomycin, given in individual doses of 8–10 mg/m^2 and at 4- to 6-week intervals, is optimally given preoperatively a maximum of 3 times; cisplatin 90–120 mg/m^2 is given over 20–120 min, not fractionated over 2 or more days; and vinblastine is given either repeatedly with weekly dosing or as a continuous infusion over 6–7 days. With vinblastine given either weekly or as a continuous infusion the duration of each MVP course is protracted and spans weeks.

Using these features of dose and schedule, results with neoadjuvant MVP are presented in table 5. Response rates with primary MVP are remarkably similar among the four series and are comparable despite the significant proportion of patients with stage IIIB disease included in the Penrose series and in the study by Henriquez et al. [23]. In the three series with surgical resection as an objective, 50–60% of all patients entered were resected following MVP. The median as well as 3-year survivals are similar in all four series, despite the predominant use in the Penrose series of radiotherapy rather than surgery for consolidation. Further, the 23% 6-year survival in the Penrose series indicates the potential for truly prolonged disease control with neoadjuvant MVP.

The significance of neoadjuvant MVP can perhaps best be appreciated by comparing consecutive series at Memorial Sloan-Kettering in which patients with stage IIIA, clinically evident N2 disease were managed in previous years with local therapy alone versus results obtained with neoadjuvant MVP. While Martini et al. [67], without primary MVP, were able to resect only 18% of such patients and reported a 3-year survival of 9% following attempted resection, brachytherapy, and postoperative external-beam radiation therapy, Pisters et al. [19] and Gralla [20] reported a 60% (44/73) resection rate and 26% 3-year survival with primary MVP, attempted resection, and postoperative thoracic irradiation.

Although it is apparent that the majority of patients entered in neoadjuvant trials are still succumbing to NSCLC, the first-generation studies shown in table 5 indicate an improvement over past experience. With conventional radiotherapy alone for this stage of disease, median and 3-year survivals are approximately 8 months and 6%, respectively [59]. It is in the neoadjuvant setting with locoregionally advanced disease that significant improvements in survival are currently achievable.

Lung Toxicity with Mitomycin

In the Penrose experience [22] lung injury was the most significant problem encountered with neoadjuvant therapy. Mitomycin has long been associated with lung toxicity [68, 69]. A large body of evidence suggests that mitomycin-induced lung injury, as well as mitomycin-associated hemolytic-uremic syndrome (HUS), are the result of vascular, more specifically, endothelial injury mediated by free-radical oxygen [70–73]. Fibrin and platelet thrombi have been frequently observed within pulmonary and renal arterioles and capillaries of patients with pulmonary and renal toxicity following treatment with mitomycin. This frequency, along with the pathogenetic significance of such thrombi, has led to the description of mitomycin-associated injury as a form of thrombotic microangiopathy (TMA) [74, 75].

Clinical syndromes resulting from mitomycin-associated TMA include HUS [76]; HUS and noncardiogenic pulmonary edema with or without blood-product transfusion [77–79]; HUS with adult respiratory-distress syndrome [78]; acute reversible bronchospasm [80, 81]; acute reversible or irreversible noncardiogenic pulmonary edema [82, 83]; acute noncardiogenic pulmonary edema with subsequent persistent respiratory failure and pathologic findings of diffuse alveolar damage-interstitial pneumonitis fibrosis (DAD-IPF) [78, 84]; and chronic progressive respiratory failure with DAD-IPF [68, 69, 85]. Rather than representing distinctly separate entities, the syndromes can be seen as overlapping segments of a spectrum of drug-induced vascular injury [86].

The large majority of mitomycin-associated lung toxicity occurs in patients receiving mitomycin in combination chemotherapy, in patients receiving mitomycin after failing initial chemotherapy, or in patients undergoing thoracic radiotherapy and/or pulmonary resection in addition to mitomycin. As of 1990 only 3 cases of interstitial fibrosis in patients given mitomycin alone have been reported [87]. Combination therapy with fluorouracil has been most often associated with the occurrence of lung toxicity [87]. Doxorubicin, well known to produce cardiac toxicity through free-radical oxygen [88], may augment mitomycin-associated vascular injury by the same mechanism. Vinca alkaloids have also been implicated in numerous laboratory and clinical studies. In vitro studies demonstrate that single-agent vinblastine produces endothelial cell disruption [89], and vindesine and concurrent thoracic radiotherapy have been associated with severe pulmonary interstitial fibrosis [90]. Numerous reports also have described acute bronchospasm and/or noncardiogenic pulmonary edema with potential progression to fatal respiratory failure with DAD-IPF following vinca alkaloid administration in patients previously treated with mitomycin as well as in patients receiving concurrent mitomycin and vinca alkaloids [80–84]. Furthermore, cisplatin and vinblastine, in combination with bleomycin but in the absence of mitomycin, have been associated with a variety of vascular complications including HUS [91–95]. Single-agent carboplatin also has produced fatal thrombotic thrombocytopenic purpura [96]. Thus, within the MVP combination, vinblastine and cisplatin appear to augment the potential of mitomycin for TMA, including overt lung toxicity.

To potentially reduce vascular injury, and to reduce the inflammatory-fibrotic response to that injury, intravenous dexamethasone preceding mitomycin began to be studied at Penrose Hospital in 1983 [22]. From 1981 through 1986, MPV was studied in 86 subjects, including patients with stage IV NSCLC treated with MPV alone, patients with stage III disease treated with neoadjuvant MPV, as well as those managed with MPV after failing primary surgery or thoracic irradiation. All 86 patients are categorized in table 6 according to specifics of treatment, including dose of dexamethasone premedication. The initial 25 patients received no corticosteroids, the subsequent 19 were given dexamethasone 7–9 mg prior to each dose of mitomycin, and the 42 patients treated thereafter received dexamethasone 10–12 mg prior to each mitomycin dose. Factors potentially contributing to lung injury, such as severity of underlying COPD (expressed as FEV_1/FVC), extent of thoracic irradiation or lung resection, and cumulative mitomycin dose are shown in table 6 and are equivalent among all three groups.

Table 6. Dexamethasone prophylaxis of mitomycin-induced lung injury: patient characteristics

	Dexamethasone, mg					
	0		7–9		10–12	
MPV alone						
No. Patients (total observations)[1]	7	(13)[2]	5	(13)[2]	21	(30)[2]
Clinical features						
Age, years	60	(36–77)	64	(47–79)	62	(44–85)
Pretherapy FEV_1/FVC (%)	74	(60–84)	65	(37–83)	64	(35–81)
Mitomycin total dose (mg/m^2)	31	(21–51)	38	(27–51)	32	(18–65)
MPV and lung irradiation						
Patients, n	9		11		13	
Clinical features						
Age, years	63	(45–77)	67	(54–78)	60	(46–75)
Pretherapy FEV_1/FVC (%)	76	(47–88)	64	(37–82)	65	(48–80)
Mitomycin total dose (mg/m^2)	24	(14–38)	33	(27–41)	34	(27–45)
RT portal area (cm^2)						
First field	163	(96–306)	144	(72–225)	169	(94–374)
Second field	32	(0–68)	30	(0–75)	36	(0–115)
Total	193	(96–329)	159	(96–288)	194	(94–347)
Fields, n	3.0	(2–6)	3.2	(2–6)	3.4	(2–8)
Gy administered						
First field	53.53	(39.6–66)	47.19	(25.67–66.0)	45.15	(27–60)
Second field	3.86	(0–19.8)	7.77	(0–25.67)	9.7	(0–37.4)
Total	57.4	(50–66)	54.51	(30.00–66)	54.91	(45.20–64.40)
MPV and lung resection						
Patients, n	9		3		8	
Clinical features						
Age, years	54	(26–73)	61	(51–72)	55	(27–78)
Pretherapy FEV_1/FVC (%)	70	(55–83)	80	(72–85)	76	(64–82)
Mitomycin total dose (mg/m^2)	36	(26–48)	39	(36–46)	32	(20–45)
Extent of resection[3]	2.3	(1–4)	2.3	(1–3)	2.3	(1–4)
Combined therapy[4]						
Patients, n	18		14		21	
Clinical features						
Age, years	59	(26–77)	65	(51–78)	58	(27–78)
Pretherapy FEV_1/FVC (%)	73	(47–88)	67	(37–85)	68	(48–82)
Mitomycin total dose (mg/m^2)	31	(14–48)	34	(27–46)	33	(20–45)
Total patients	25		19		42	
Clinical features						
Age, years	58	(26–77)	65	(47–79)	61	(27–85)
Pretherapy FEV_1/FVC (%)	72	(47–88)	67	(37–83)	67	(35–81)
Mitomycin total dose (mg/m^2)	31	(14–51)	36	(27–51)	33	(17–65)

1 Data expressed as mean (range).
2 Patients receiving MPV only and those receiving MPV prior to radiotherapy or surgery.
3 1 = 1 lobe or less; 2 = 2 lobes; 3 = pneumonectomy; 4 = pneumonectomy and radiotherapy.
4 Mitomycin, cisplatin, continuous infusion vinblastine and resection or radiotherapy.

Table 7. Dexamethasone prophylaxis of mitomycin-induced lung injury

	Dexa-methasone 0 mg	p value[1]	Dexa-methasone 10–12 mg	p value[1]	Dexa-methasone 7–9 mg
MPV alone					
Patients (total observations)[2]	7 (13)		21 (30)		5 (13)
Toxic syndrome[3]	2	0.086	0	–	0
Died, DAD-IPF[4] minimal or no NSCLC	1	–	0	–	0
MPV and lung irradiation					
Patients	9		13		11
Toxic syndrome[3]	4	–	2	–	3
Died, DAD-IPF[4] minimal or no NSCLC	1	–	0	–	2
MPV and lung resection					
Patients	9		8		3
Toxic syndrome[3]	4	0.053	0	0.27	1
Died, DAD-IPF[4] minimal or no NSCLC	3	0.2	0	0.27	1
Combined therapy[5] – total					
Patients	18		21		14
Toxic syndrome[3]	8	0.016	2	0.15	4
Died, DAD-IPF[4] minimal or no NSCLC	4	0.037	0	0.060	3
Total patients	25		42		19
Toxic syndrome[3]	10	0.00050	2	0.069	4
Died, DAD-IPF[4] minimal or no NSCLC	5	0.0055	0	0.027	3

1 Fisher's exact test, significant at 0.05 level.
2 Patients receiving MPV only plus those receiving MPV prior to radiotherapy or surgery.
3 Dyspnea, hypoxemia, chest X-ray consistent with mitomycin lung injury, corticosteroids.
4 Diffuse alveolar damage, interstitial pneumonitis fibrosis.
5 Mitomycin, cisplatin, continuous infusion vinblastine and resection or radiotherapy.

Results of corticosteroid prophylaxis are shown in table 7. In the group receiving MPV alone and without dexamethasone, overt lung injury developed in 2 patients, 1 of whom died. In contrast, no patient treated with MPV alone but with dexamethasone 7–9 mg or 10–12 mg given prior to each dose of mitomycin developed clinically evident toxicity.

With combined-modality therapy, patients who received the smaller dose of dexamethasone encountered toxicity approximately equivalent to that observed in those receiving no prophylaxis, and both groups experienced more problems than did patients given dexamethasone 10–12 mg. Overall, the administration of dexamethasone 10–12 mg prior to each mitomycin dose was associated with a significantly reduced incidence of respiratory complications (table 7).

While dexamethasone premedication reduces the frequency and severity of treatment-associated complications, the protection is relative and not absolute. Additional mitomycin or chemotherapeutic agents that potentiate lung injury, more extensive surgical resection, or expanded radiotherapy portals, may override the protective effect of corticosteroids. Two of 13 patients in the Penrose neoadjuvant series received dexamethasone 10–12 mg as prophylaxis prior to mitomycin but developed reversible toxicity following consolidation with thoracic radiotherapy. Consistent with this experience, a report by Hoelzer et al. [97] describes the development of reversible acute respiratory failure in 2 of 33 patients treated with MVP alone, despite premedication with dexamethasone (dose unspecified) as an antiemetic.

Table 8. Response to MPV with and without intravenous dexamethasone preceding mitomycin.

	Dexamethasone 4–9 mg		Dexamethasone 0		Dexamethasone 10–12 mg
Stage III	5/12		7/8		8/15
Stage IV	0/4		4/6		3/15
	—	p value*	—	p value*	—
Total Responders[+]	5/16	<0.025	11/14	<0.025	11/30

* Cochran corrected Chi-square.
[+] Complete or partial response by standard criteria.

Unfortunately, corticosteroid premedication produces global anti-inflammatory effects, and administration of these agents appears to diminish the antineoplastic effect of mitomycin. Sixty of the total 86 patients at Penrose Hospital in whom dexamethasone prophylaxis of lung toxicity was studied (see above) were also evaluable for tumor response with and without dexamethasone (table 8). The response rate in patients not given dexamethasone was superior to that in patients receiving dexamethasone prior to mitomycin. While the number of patients treated without dexamethasone was small, and the response rate without dexamethasone was higher than usually reported, a clear difference in response rates was observed.

Guidelines for Mitomycin Use

Consideration of the following points will help reduce the frequency and severity of mitomycin-associated complications.

Cumulative and Individual Dose of Mitomycin

Mitomycin-associated toxicity is dose-dependent. Although there is, in abstract form, a single case report [98] of fatal HUS following mitomycin 5 mg in conjunction with doxorubicin and vincristine, mitomycin-associated TMA appears to be distinctly uncommon with cumulative mitomycin doses of <30 mg/m^2. Verwey et al. [99], reviewing total mitomycin doses in 88 case reports of mitomycin-associated renal toxicity, including HUS, found the median cumulative dose to be 60 mg/m^2, with no renal toxicity occurring in patients receiving <30 mg/m^2. Only 9 of 83 cases (11%) of mitomycin-associated HUS reported in the HUS Registry [77] occurred following <60 mg total dose. Verweij et al. [100], reviewing the literature, reported that the median cumulative dose in patients developing overt pulmonary interstitial fibrosis was 50 mg/m^2 (20–200 mg/m^2). Only 2 patients developed overt lung injury with a cumulative dose of 20–30 mg/m^2. Mitomycin total dose is thus a significant variable in the development of toxicity.

As mentioned earlier, sensitivity of NSCLC to mitomycin-containing combination chemotherapy becomes evident within the initial 2 courses, and the maximum clinically discernable tumor reduction occurs within a total of 3 courses. The risk of toxicity increases – and the likelihood of significant benefit decreases – with cumulative doses greater than 30 mg/m^2 or with an absolute cumulative total dose exceeding 60 mg.

Intervals between Courses

Studies of mitomycin administered at 3-week intervals reveal increased toxicity over those with longer intervals between courses [101, 102]. With mitomycin 8–10 mg/m^2 and cisplatin 100–120 mg/m^2, patients require at least 4 weeks between the initial and 2nd cycles, and at least 6 weeks between the 2nd and 3rd courses. With neoadjuvant approaches, patients require a minimum of 7 weeks from beginning the 3rd course to the start of local consolidation.

Prophylactic Corticosteroids

Although administration of corticosteroids prior to mitomycin provides relative protection from toxicity, corticosteroid premedication reduces the antineoplastic effect of mitomycin (see above). Nothing is easy in the management of NSCLC. Steroid prophylaxis appears more advantageous prior to the oxidative stresses of thoracotomy.

Perioperative Management

Preoperative communication with the anesthesiologist and surgeon is essential. While the specifics of intraoperative management depend on developments that unfold during thoracotomy, and must therefore be individualized, the likelihood of postoperative respiratory complications appears to be reduced by the following measures: (1) giving methylprednisolone 250 mg i.v. just prior to surgery; (2) minimizing the oxygen fraction of inspired gas (FIO_2) (This measure was originally described by Goldiner et al. [103] with preoperative bleomycin and Franklin et al. [104] with preoperative mitomycin and thoracic radiotherapy. While the lower the oxygen content the better, an FIO_2 of 35–45% has been adequate following preoperative corticosteroids); (3) minimizing use of intraoperative i.v. fluids to avoid pulmonary edema secondary to a 'leaky' alveolar-capillary membrane (Use colloids in place of crystalloids); (4) avoiding intraoperative erythrocyte transfusion. Microangiopathic hemolytic anemia is to be carefully excluded preoperatively. If needed, transfusions can be carried out cautiously preoperatively [105]; (5) avoiding pneumonectomy, if possible [106].

Cessation of Smoking

As a result of pulmonary-specific inflammatory and metabolic changes related to smoking, patients who continue to use tobacco may be predisposed to treatment-induced lung injury.

Patient Assessment

Patients need to be evaluated repeatedly regarding development of the following symptoms or signs: (1) dyspnea, particularly dyspnea with minor exertion; (2) inspiratory rales and/or pleural rub; (3) a new, unexplained roentgenographic infiltrate or effusion; and (4) otherwise unexplained thrombocytopenia, particularly gradually progressive thrombocytopenia unrelated to chemotherapy. 'Disseminated intravascular platelet adhesion and aggregation' has been described as central to the pathophysiology of HUS and thrombotic thrombocytopenic purpura [107]. In the Penrose experience [22], 8 of 16 patients developing overt lung injury were also thrombocytopenic, but without hemolysis or renal insufficiency. Platelet counts tended to fall or rise in association with worsening or improving lung function. Platelet transfusions to thrombocytopenic patients with marginal respiratory function tended to worsen lung function.

Development of the aforementioned symptoms or signs requires that all further treatment, including vinca alkaloids and cisplatin, be withheld pending an explanation. Following completion of treatment, patients need to be followed for potential toxicity for at least 12–18 months. Neoadjuvant mitomycin should not be administered to patients who cannot be closely followed.

In patients suspected of developing early treatment-induced injury but who do not have overt symptoms or signs, minimal conservative management includes antiplatelet therapy with dipyridamole and low-dose aspirin, withholding of all chemotherapy (including vinca alkaloids and cisplatin) and thoracic radiotherapy, and aggressive nontransfusion of erythrocytes or platelets.

Remain Cautious: There Are No Absolutes

In patients who respond well to initial mitomycin-containing treatment, avoid the temptation to proceed more quickly with additional intervention. Most patients who develop various forms of mitomycin-associated toxicity have been noted to be either responding well to treatment, in clinical remission, or to have no objective evidence of carcinoma. Development of lung injury or HUS is much less common in patients with clinical evidence of progressive cancer [22, 75, 78, 105].

Avoid the temptation to use everything – chemotherapy, radiotherapy, and surgery.

Patients who have undergone prior lung resection or have received radiotherapy and who subsequently receive mitomycin at the time of relapse require the same precautions as those prospectively treated with mitomycin in combined-modality therapy.

Three courses of MVP prior to 50–60 Gy of conventionally fractionated thoracic radiotherapy is potentially hazardous. This approach is not encouraged in the absence of specific prophylaxis against lung injury or in the absence of measures to detect patients with early subclinical toxic effects. All of these factors must be embodied within an investigational protocol.

Conclusion

Achievement of even limited therapeutic goals in advanced NSCLC requires significant intervention, and therefore significant patient and physician commitment. For the medical oncologist this entails considerable time, thought, and close patient observation. Attempts to 'short-cut' patient management, to render the treatment of NSCLC more 'efficient' through the use of low-dose, convenient therapy have not led to further tumor regression, and have not improved patient survival or quality of life. While reports of the highest rates of objective regression of advanced NSCLC have included mitomycin in appropriate schedule and cumulative dose, weekly bolus or infusion vinblastine, and higher-dose cisplatin, responses to chemotherapy alone tend to be brief. For this reason application of a second, potentially non-cross-resistant, therapeutic modality to the complete extent of initially demonstrable disease is essential. Thus, the impact of mitomycin-containing chemotherapy is greatest in stage III disease where the advantages of greater intrinsic chemotherapy sensitivity, greater patient tolerance, and potential for surgery and/or radiation therapy in addition to chemotherapy appears to improve survival in comparison with traditional radiotherapy alone.

Significant toxicity has been documented with mitomycin-containing therapy and, as a result, this agent frequently has been avoided. It is now clear, however, that the well-described complications with which mitomycin has been associated are primarily related to cumulative dose and schedule of the drug, and related as well to other chemotherapeutic agents and therapeutic modalities with which mitomycin has been combined. Fortunately, practical guidelines for more effective use of mitomycin have evolved, allowing for realization of the vital contribution of mitomycin to therapeutic approaches to the management of NSCLC. Future studies are needed to determine more sensitive and specific monitors of early, subclinical chemotherapy-induced vascular injury, as well as to establish more precise means to prevent subsequent overt toxicity.

References

1 Kris M, Cohen E, Gralla R: An analysis of 134 phase II trials in non-small cell lung cancer (NSCLC). Proceedings of the IVth World Conference on Lung Cancer (abstract). Toronto, Canada, 1985;4:39.

2 Gralla R, Casper ES, Kelsen DP, et al: Cisplatin and vindesine combination chemotherapy for advanced carcinoma of the lung: A randomized trial investigating two dosing schedules. Ann Intern Med 1981;96:414–420.

3 Kris MG, Gralla RJ, Wertheim MS, et al: Trial of the combination of mitomycin, vindesine and cisplatin in patients with advanced non-small cell lung cancer. Cancer Treat Rep 1986; 70:1091–1096.

4 Rapp E, Pater JL, Willan A, et al: Chemotherapy can prolong survival in patients with advanced non-small lung cancer: Report of a Canadian multicenter randomized trial. J Clin Oncol 1988;6:633–641.

5 Dillman RO, Seagren SL, Propert KJ, et al: A randomized trial of induction chemotherapy plus high-dose radiation versus radiation alone in stage III non-small cell lung cancer. N Engl J Med 1990;323:940–945.

6 Martini N, Kris MG, Gralla RJ: The effects of preoperative chemotherapy on the resectability of non-small cell lung carcinoma with mediastinal lymph node metastases (N2M0). Ann Thorac Surg 1988;45:370–379.

7 O'Connell JP, Kris MG, Gralla RJ, et al: Frequency and prognostic importance of pretreatment clinical characteristics in patients with advanced non-small cell lung cancer treated with combination chemotherapy. J Clin Oncol 1986;4:1604–1614.

8 Paesmans M, Donnadieu N, Sculier JP: Increased response rate in patients with non-metastatic non-small cell lung cancer (NSCLC): A meta analysis of the literature. Proc Am Soc Clin Oncol 1990;9:251 (abstract).

9 Bonomi P: Brief overview of combination chemotherapy in non-small cell lung cancer. Semin Oncol 1986;13(suppl 3):89–91.

10 Blum R, Cooper J, Schmidt A, et al: Cisplatin and vinblastine chemotherapy for metastatic non-small cell carcinoma followed by radiation in patients with regional disease. Cancer Treat Rep 1986;70:333–337.

11 Fukuoka M, Masuda N, Furuse K, et al: A randomized trial in inoperable non-small cell lung cancer: Vindesine and cisplatin versus mitomycin, vindesine and cisplatin versus etoposide and cisplatin alternating with vindesine and mitomycin. J Clin Oncol 1991;9:606–613.

12 Samson MK, Comis RL, Baker LH, et al: Mitomycin C in advanced adenocarcinoma and large cell carcinoma of the lung. Cancer Treat Rep 1978;62:163–165.

13 Ruckdeschel JC, Mehta CR, Salazar OM, et al: Chemotherapy for inoperable non-small cell bronchogenic carcinoma: EST 2575, generation II. Cancer Treat Rep 1981;65:965–972.

14 Koons LS, Catalano RB, Harris DT: Mitomycin C in epidermoid cancer of the lung; in Carter SK, Crooke ST (eds): Mitomycin C: Current Status and New Developments. New York, Academic Press, 1979, pp 189–192.

15 Niell HB, Griffin JP, Hunter RF, et al: Combination versus sequential single agent chemotherapy in the treatment of patients with advanced non-small cell lung cancer. Med Pediatr Oncol 1989;17:69–75.

16 Veeder M, Jett J, Su JQ, et al: A phase III trial of mitomycin C alone versus mitomycin C, vinblastine, and cisplatin for metastatic squamous cell lung carcinoma. Cancer 1992;70: 2281–2287.

17 Albain K, Crowley J, LeBlanc M, et al: Does cisplatin (DDP)-based therapy improve survival in extensive non-small cell lung cancer (NSCLC)? Southwest Oncology Group (SWOG) studies. Proc Am Soc Clin Oncol 1990;9:227 (abstract).

18 Bunn PA: The expanding role of cisplatin in the treatment of non-small cell lung cancer. Semin Oncol 1989;16(4):10–21.

19 Pisters KMW, Kris MG, Gralla RJ, et al: Preoperative chemotherapy in stage III non-small cell lung cancer: An analysis of a trial in patients with clinically apparent mediastinal node involvement; in Salmon SE (ed): Adjuvant Therapy of Cancer, ed 6. Philadelphia, WB Saunders, 1990, pp 133–137.

20 Gralla RJ: Preoperative and adjuvant chemotherapy in non-small cell lung cancer. Semin Oncol 1988;15(suppl 7):8–12.

21 Burkes R, Ginsberg R, Sheperd F, et al: Induction chemotherapy with mitomycin, vindesine, and cisplatin for stage III unresectable non-small cell lung cancer: Results of the Toronto phase II trial. J Clin Oncol 1992;10:580–586.

22 Spain R: Neoadjuvant mitomycin-C, cisplatin and infusion vinblastine in locally and regionally advanced non-small cell lung cancer: Problems and progress from the perspective of long-term follow-up. Semin Oncol 1988;15 (suppl 4):6–15.

23 Henriquez I, Galindo L, Rebollo J, et al: Neoadjuvant chemotherapy (NAC) with cisplatin (CDDP), vindesine (VDS), and mitomycin-C (MMC) in locally advanced non-small cell lung cancer (NSCLC) (abstract). Proc Am Soc Clin Oncol 1990;9:227.
24 Hayes DM, Cvitkovic E, Golbey RB, et al: High dose cisplatinum diamminedichloride: Amelioration of renal toxicity by mannitol diuresis. Cancer 1977;39:1372–1381.
25 Kris MG, Gralla RJ, Tyson LB, et al: Improved control of cisplatin-induced emesis with high-dose metoclopramide and with combinations of metoclopramide, dexamethasone and diphenhydramine. Results of consecutive trials in 255 patients. Cancer 1985;55:527–534.
26 Einhorn LE, Nagy C, Werner K, Finn AL: Ondansetron: A new antiemetic for patients receiving cisplatin. J Clin Oncol 1990;8:731–735.
27 Whittington RM, Close HP: Clinical experience with mitomycin C (NSC-26980). Cancer Chemother Rep 1970;54/3:195–198.
28 Rosso R, Ardizzone A, Salvati F, et al: Etoposide vs. etoposide and cisplatin in the treatment of advanced non-small cell lung cancer: A FONICAP randomized study. Semin Oncol 1988;15(suppl 7):49–51.
29 Klastersky J, Sculier JP, Bureau G, et al: Cisplatin versus cisplatin plus etoposide in the treatment of advanced non-small cell lung cancer. J Clin Oncol 1989;7:1087–1092.
30 Gatzemeier V, Heckmayr M, Neuhauss R, et al: Phase III studies with carboplatin in non-small cell lung cancer. Semin Oncol 1990;17/1 (suppl 2):25–31.
31 Johnson DH, Einhorn LH, Bartolucci A, et al: Thoracic radiotherapy does not prolong survival in patients with locally advanced unresectable non-small cell lung cancer. Ann Intern Med 1990;113:33–38.
32 Elliot JA, Ahmedzai S, Hole D, et al: Vindesine and cisplatin combination chemotherapy compared with vindesine as a single agent in the management of non-small cell lung cancer: A randomized study. Eur J Cancer Clin Oncol 1984;20:1025–1032.
33 Gralla RJ, Raphael BG, Golbeu RB, et al: Phase II evaluation of vindesine in patients with non-small cell carcinoma of the lung. Cancer Treat Rep 1979;63:1343–1346.
34 Bonomi PD, Finkelstein DM, Ruckdeschel JC, et al: Combination chemotherapy versus single agents followed by combination chemotherapy in stage IV non-small cell lung cancer: A study of the Eastern Cooperative Oncology Group. J Clin Oncol 1989;7:1602–1613.
35 Olver IN, Donehower RC, van Echo DA, et al: Phase II trial of carboplatin in non-small cell lung cancer. Cancer Treat Rep 1986;70:421–422.
36 Kreisman H, Ginsberg S, Propert KJ, et al: Carboplatin or iproplatin in advanced non-small cell lung cancer: A Cancer and Leukemia Group B Study. Cancer Treat Rep 1987;71:1049–1052.
37 Kramer BS, Birch R, Greco A, et al: Randomized phase II evaluation of iproplatin (CHIP) and carboplatin (CBDCA) in lung cancer: A Southeastern Cancer Study Group trial. Am J Clin Oncol 1988;11:643–645.
38 Loehrer PJ, Birch R, Kramer BS, et al: Ifosfamide plus N-acetylcysteine in the treatment of small cell and non-small cell carcinoma of the lung: A Southeastern Cancer Study Group trial. Cancer Treat Rep 1986;70:919–920.
39 Livingston R: Discussion. Semin Oncol 1988;15(suppl 7):62–70.
40 Casper ES, Gralla RS, Kelsen DP, et al: Phase II study of high dose *cis*-dichlorodiammineplatinum (II) in the treatment of non-small cell lung cancer. Cancer Treat Rep 1979;63:2107–2109.
41 Bhuchar VK, Lanzotti VJ: High-dose cisplatin for lung cancer. Cancer Treat Rep 1982;66:375–376.
42 Gandara DR, Tanaka MT, Crowley J, et al: Comparison of standard-dose cisplatin, high-dose cisplatin and high-dose cisplatin plus mitomycin in metastatic non-small cell lung cancer (abstract). Proc Am Soc Clin Oncol 1991;10:246.
43 Crino L, Darwish S, Corgna E, et al: Treatment of advanced non-small cell lung cancer (NSCLC): The 'Umbria' cooperative study. Semin Oncol 1988;15/6(suppl 7):52–55.
44 Walters RS, Frye D, Buzdar A, et al: A randomized trial of two dosage schedules of mitomycin-C in advanced breast carcinoma. Cancer 1992;69:476–481.
45 Creech RH, Catalano RB, Shah MK, et al: An effective, low dose mitomycin regimen for hormonal and chemotherapy refractory patients with metastatic breast cancer. Cancer 1983;51:1034–1040.
46 Krook JE, Jett JR, Fleming TR, et al: A controlled evaluation of combined 5-fluorouracil, doxorubicin and mitomycin C (FAM) for the treatment of advanced non-small cell lung cancer. J Clin Oncol 1985;3(6):842–848.
47 Eagan RT, Frytak S, Creagan E, et al: Differing response rates and survival between squamous and nonsquamous non-small cell lung cancer. Am J Clin Oncol 1986;9:249–254.
48 Luedke D, Luedke S, Martello O, et al: Response of non-small cell lung cancer (NSCLC) to vindesine (VD) and mitomycin-C (MITO): A Southeastern Cancer Study Group pilot study (abstract). Proc Am Soc Clin Oncol 1983;3:190.
49 Luedke DW, Einhorn L, Omura GA, et al: Randomized comparison of two combination regimens versus minimal chemotherapy in non-small cell lung cancer: A Southeastern Cancer Study Group trial. J Clin Oncol 1990;8:886–891.
50 Kris MG, Gralla RJ, Kelsen DP, et al: Trial of vindesine plus mitomycin in stage III non-small cell lung cancer: An active regimen for outpatient treatment. Chest 1985;87:368–372.
51 Weick JK, Rainey JM, Livingston RB, et al: Treatment of non-small cell bronchogenic carcinoma with vinblastine and mitomycin: A Southwest Oncology Group study. Cancer Treat Rep 1985;69:583–585.
52 Shinkai T, Saijo N, Tominaga K, et al: Comparison of vindesine plus cisplatin or vindesine plus mitomycin in the treatment of advanced non-small cell lung cancer. Cancer Treat Rep 1985;69:945–951.
53 Sculier JP, Klastersky J, Dumont JP, et al: Combination chemotherapy with mitomycin and vindesine in advanced non-small cell lung cancer: A pilot study by the Lung Cancer Working Party (Belgium). Cancer Treat Rep 1986;70:773–775.
54 Gatzemeier V, Heckmayr M, Hossfeld DK, et al: A randomized trial with mitomycin-C/ifosfamide versus mitomycin-C/vindesine versus cisplatin/etoposide in advanced non-small cell lung cancer. Am J Clin Oncol 1991;14:405–411.
55 Gralla RJ, Kris MG, Burke MT, et al: The influence of the addition of mitomycin (M) to vindesine (V) plus cisplatin (P) in a random assignment trial in 120 patients with non-small cell lung cancer (NSCLC) (abstract). Proc Am Soc Clin Oncol 1986;5:182.
56 Roswit B, Patno ME, Rapp R, et al: The survival of patients with inoperable lung cancer: A large scale randomized study of radiation therapy versus placebo. Radiology 1968;90:688–697.
57 Komaki R, Cox JD, Hartz AJ, et al: Characteristics of long-term survivors after treatment for inoperable carcinoma of the lung. Am J Clin Oncol 1985;8:362–370.
58 Mountain C: A new international staging system. Chest 1986;89:2255–2335.
59 Perez CA, Stanley K, Grundy G, et al: Impact of irradiation technique and tumor extent in tumor control and survival of patients with unresectable non-oat cell carcinoma of the lung: Report by the Radiation Therapy Oncology Group. Cancer1982;50:1091–1099.
60 Perez CA: Non-small cell carcinoma of the lung: Dose-time parameters. Cancer Treat Symp 1985;2:131–142.
61 Mountain CF, McMurtrey MJ, Frazier OH, et al: Present status of postoperative adjuvant therapy for lung cancer. Cancer Bull 1980;32:108–121.
62 Martini N, Flehinger B, Zaman MB, et al: Results of resection in non-oat cell carcinoma of the lung with mediastinal lymph node metastases. Ann Surg 1983;198:386–397.
63 Perez CA, Rubin P, Frances M, et al: Patterns of failure in localized unresectable non-oat cell carcinoma of the lung treated by radiation therapy (abstract). Proc Am Soc Clin Oncol 1984;20:23.
64 The Lung Cancer Study Group: Effects of postoperative mediastinal radiation on completely resected stage II and stage III epidermoid cancer of the lung. N Engl J Med 1986;315:1377–1381.

65 Goldie JH: Scientific basis for adjuvant and primary (neoadjuvant) chemotherapy. Semin Oncol 1987;14:1–7.
66 Nelson RL, Dyla RW, Root MA: Comparative pharmacokinetics of vindesine, vincristine and vinblastine in patients with cancer. Cancer Treat Rev 1980;7(suppl 1):17–24.
67 Martini N, Flehinger BJ: The role of surgery in N2 lung cancer. Surg Clin North Amer 1987; 67(5):1037–1049.
68 Simasota Y, Baba K, Watanabe S: Pulmonary lesions produced by antitumor drugs. Studies on autopsy cases. Jpn J Cancer Clin 1971;17: 21–34.
69 Orwoll ES, Kiessling PH, Patterson JR: Interstitial pneumonia from mitomycin. Ann Intern Med 1978;89:352–353.
70 Spain RC, Whittlesey D: Respiratory emergencies in patients with cancer. Semin Oncol 1989;16(6):471–489.
71 Pritsos CA, Sartorelli AC: Generation of reactive oxygen radicals through bioactivation of mitomycin antibiotics. Cancer Res 1986;436: 3528–3532.
72 Cattell V: Mitomycin induced hemolytic uremic kidney. An experimental model in the rat. Am J Pathol 1985;121:88–95.
73 Trush MA, Mimwaugh EG, Ginsberg E, et al: Studies on the in vitro interaction of mitomycin-C, nitrofurantoin, and paraquat with pulmonary microsomes: Stimulation of reactive oxygen dependent lipid peroxidation. Biochem Pharmacol 1982;31:805–814.
74 Murgo AJ: Thrombotic microangiopathy in the cancer patient including those induced by chemotherapeutic agents. Semin Hematol 1987;24:161–177.
75 Murgo AJ: Cancer and chemotherapy associated thrombotic microangiopathy; in Kaplan BS, Trompeter RS, Moake JL (eds). The Hemolytic-Uremic Syndrome/Thrombotic Thrombocytopenic Purpura. New York, Dekker, 1992.
76 Cantrell JE, Phillips TRM, Schein PS: Carcinoma associated hemolytic-uremic syndrome: A complication of mitomycin-C chemotherapy. J Clin Oncol 1985;3:723–734.
77 Lesesne JB, Rothschild N, Erickson B, et al: Cancer associated hemolytic-uremic syndrome: Analysis of 85 cases from a national registry. J Clin Oncol 1989;7:781–789.
78 Sheldon R, Slaughter D: A syndrome of microangiopathic hemolytic anemia, renal impairment, and pulmonary edema in chemotherapy treated patients with adenocarcinoma. Cancer 1986;58:1428–1436.
79 Jolivet J, Giroux L, Lauris S, et al: Microangiopathic hemolytic anemia, renal failure and noncardiogenic pulmonary edema: A chemotherapy induced syndrome. Cancer Treat Rep 1983;67:429–434.
80 Kris MG, Pablo D, Gralla RJ, et al: Dyspnea following vinblastine or vindesine administration in patients receiving mitomycin plus vinca alkaloid combination therapy. Cancer Treat Rep 1984;68:1029–1031.
81 Luedke D, McLaughlin T, Daughaday C, et al: Mitomycin-C and vindesine associated pulmonary toxicity with variable clinical expression. Cancer 1985;55:542–545.
82 Israel RH, Olson JP: Pulmonary edema associated with intravenous vinblastine. JAMA 1978;240:1585.
83 Rao SX, Ramaswany G, Levin M, et al: Fatal acute respiratory failure after vinblastine-mitomycin therapy for lung cancer. Arch Intern Med 1985;145:1905–1907.
84 Konits PH, Aisner H, Sutherland JC, et al: Possible pulmonary toxicity secondary to vinblastine. Cancer 1982;50:2771–2774.
85 Buzdar AU, Legha SS, Luna MA, et al: Pulmonary toxicity of mitomycin. Cancer 1980; 45:236–244.
86 Remuzzi G: Nephrology forum: HUS and TTP: Variable expression of a single entity. Kidney Int 1987;32:292–308.
87 Twohig KS, Matthay RA: Pulmonary effects of cytotoxic agents other than bleomycin. Clin Chest Med 1990;11/1:31–54.
88 Doroshow JH: Role of reactive oxygen production in doxorubicin cardiac toxicity; in Hacker MP, Lazo JS, Tritton TR (eds): Organ Directed Toxicities of Anticancer Drugs. Boston, Nijhoff, 1987, pp 31–40.
89 Nicolson G, Custead S: Effects of chemotherapeutic drugs on platelet and metastatic tumor cell-endothelial cell interactions as a model for assessing vascular endothelial integrity. Cancer Res 1985;45:331–336.
90 Bott SJ, Stewart FM, Prince-Fiocco MA: Interstitial lung disease associated with vindesine and radiation therapy for carcinoma of the lung. South Med J 1986;79:894–896.
91 Doll DC, List AF, Greco FA, et al: Acute vascular ischemic events after cisplatin based combination chemotherapy for germ cell tumors of the testis. Ann Intern Med 1981;95: 288–292.
92 Vogelzang NJ, Bosl GJ, Johnson K, et al: Raynaud's phenomenon: A common toxicity after combination chemotherapy for testicular cancer. Ann Intern Med 1981;95:288–292.
93 Harrell RM, Sibley R, Vogelzang NJ: Renal vascular lesions after chemotherapy with vinblastine, bleomycin and cisplatin. Am J Med 1982;73:429–433.
94 Jackson AM, Rose BD, Graff LG, et al: Thrombotic microangiopathy and renal failure associated with antineoplastic chemotherapy. Ann Intern Med 1984;101:41–44.
95 Watson PR, Guthrie TRH, Caruana RJ: Cisplatin associated hemolytic-uremic syndrome: Successful treatment with a staphylococcal protein A column. Cancer 1989;64: 1400–1403.
96 Walker RW, Rosenblum MK, Kempin SJ, et al: Carboplatin associated thrombotic microangiopathic hemolytic anemia. Cancer 1989;64:1017–1020.
97 Hoelzer KL, Harrison BR, Luedke SW, et al: Vinblastine associated pulmonary toxicity in patients receiving combination therapy with mitomycin and cisplatin. Drug Intell Clin Pharm 1986;20:287–289.
98 Khojasteh A, Reynolds RD, Garcia AR, et al: Hemolytic-uremic like syndrome following a single dose of mitomycin-C (abstract). Proc Am Soc Clin Oncol 1984;3:4.
99 Verwey J, DeVries J, Pinedo HM: Mitomycin-C induced renal toxicity, a dose-dependent side effect? Eur J Cancer Clin Oncol 1987;23 (2):195–199.
100 Verweij J, van Zantern T, Souren T, et al: Prospective study on the dose relationship of mitomycin-C induced interstitial pneumonitis. Cancer 1987;60:756–761.
101 Doyle LA, Ihde DC, Carney DN, et al: Combination chemotherapy with doxorubicin and mitomycin-C in non-small cell bronchogenic carcinoma. Severe pulmonary toxicity from q3 weekly mitomycin-C. Am J Clin Oncol 1984;7:719–724.
102 Pavy MD, Wiley EL, Abeloff MD: Hemolytic-uremic syndrome associated with mitomycin therapy. Cancer Treat Rep 1982;66:457–461.
103 Goldiner P, Carlon G, Cvitkovic E, et al: Factors influencing postoperative morbidity and mortality in patients treated with bleomycin. Br Med J 1978;i:1644–1677.
104 Franklin R, Buroker T, Vaishampayan G, et al: Combined therapies in esophageal squamous cell cancer (abstract). Proc Am Assoc Cancer Res 1979;20:223.
105 Johnston-Early A, Cohen MH, Fossick BE, et al: Treatment related diffuse interstitial pulmonary disease (DIPD). A retrospective review (abstract). Proc Am Soc Clin Oncol 1982;1:146.
106 Fowler WC, Langer CJ, Keller SM, et al: Excessive morbidity and mortality of pneumonectomy following concurrent chemotherapy (5-fluorouracil, cisplatin, etoposide) and high-dose thoracic radiation (RT) for locally advanced non-small cell lung cancer (abstract). Proc Am Soc Clin Oncol 1991;10:255.
107 Kwaan HC: Role of fibrinolysis in thrombotic thrombocytopenia purpura. Semin Hematol 1987;24/2:101–109.

Discussion

Dr. Henderson: Thinking over what's been said this morning on the treatment of lung cancer, it seems to me we are not at all certain of the contribution of the various agents used. What is the role of ifosfamide, for instance? What do the vincas add? Everybody seems to be saying that platinum is the most active agent in most regimens. If we discuss mechanism of action, do we have evidence to suggest these agents might be synergistic, or have a different mechanism of action and therefore be additive? Is there anything that should be put on the record regarding either the interactions between mitomycin and platinum or mitomycin and ifosfamide?

Dr. Cullen: There is in vitro data showing interaction among different alkylating agents. But that is not the reason any of us have put these drugs together. From my own experience, initially with just ifosfamide and mitomycin, our finding that the response rate of the combination was better than we would expect with either drug alone was rather exciting. We subsequently added cisplatin empirically for further improvement. We're a long way away, however, from knowing the biochemical injury responsible for these drugs' effects.

Dr. Gralla: Right. I think we've been most successful when we empirically build on prior results.

Dr. Henderson: Lung cancer treatment has been dominated by the CAP (cyclophosphamide/doxorubicin/cisplatin) and CAMP (cyclophosphamide/doxorubin/methotrexate/procarbazine hydrochloride) regimens. In particular, a large number of people taking care of or studying patients with lung cancer emphasize the CAP approach. Would anyone like to comment on why that might be?

Dr. Spain: At your institution in Boston, Dr. Henderson, CAP is still a favored regimen for treatment of lung cancer. But I don't think that's true across the board. CAP was the first good regimen in lung cancer and Bob Egan of the Mayo Clinic should be given a lot of credit for the good work he initiated with it. But there is no study that shows that it has any reliable efficacy. An M. D. Anderson Cancer Center study done in the 1970s found that cyclophosphamide as a single agent had only a 4% response rate. A study of vindesine versus cyclophosphamide/doxorubicin resulted in superior activity with vindesine. I can't understand why cyclophosphamide and doxorubicin remain in the regimen at all. Platinum was the effective agent in that group, with little added benefit from the others. We've also done a CAP study and had a similar response rate. However, we used high-dose platinum, and our duration of response and survival were better. The CAMP and MACC (methotrexate/doxorubicin/cyclophosphamide/CCNU) regimens have no active agents, on the other hand. I think that when they seem to have an effect it may be an issue of histology: Some of those patients may have had small cell rather than non-small cell lung cancer. Overall, you don't find too many people who subscribe to either of those regimens anymore.

Dr. Gralla: There's probably no more active single agent than mitomycin. That's an important point that people in the community do not understand. There have been few studies done, but Lucian Israel did report an extremely high response rate with mitomycin and platinum a number of years ago. Unfortunately, that experience was never followed up.

Dr. Hortobagyi: The issue of dose or dose intensity has not been addressed clearly in any of the regimens or diseases we've been discussing. Certainly, reservations about the steepness of the dose intensity curve above and beyond what is considered the clinically maximally tolerated dose are appropriate. I also believe, however, that there is a point below which an agent will no longer contribute anything to a combination. We have to be careful not to accidentally overstep this bound.

In breast cancer, platinum and several other single agents like doxorubicin have shown a correlation between dose and response, and probably even some correlation with survival. Before we go on reducing doses, I think it is important to study the question of minimal effective doses. I don't feel that this issue has been addressed in any of the studies done to date.

Dr. Henderson: Well, you've actually anticipated my last question – what studies specifically related to the use of mitomycin for lung cancer do you think should be performed? I wonder if there is such a thing as too low a dose of mitomycin? It may be a unique characteristic of this drug that there isn't a steep dose-response curve and we could, in fact, get great efficacy, particularly in combinations, with relatively low doses.

Dr. Gralla: Another potentially important avenue for future research is the value of concurrent radiation therapy and chemotherapy in non-small cell lung cancer, particularly with the combination of mitomycin and platinum. This combination was used in concurrent radiation and chemotherapy trials for gastrointestinal cancers. Unfortunately, the results were not good, perhaps because of concern over the toxicities of those individual drugs. With the relatively low doses used, median survival was mediocre and the rate of distant relapse was high. The chemotherapy was compromised in order to provide concurrent chemotherapy and radiation.

Dr. Hortobagyi: Intra-arterial use of mitomycin is another area that has not been explored much in the United States. It is probably not pertinent to lung cancer, but might be useful for pelvic malignancies and maybe even for gastric cancer. The drug is well tolerated intra-arterially and, at least anecdotally, I have seen some very dramatic responses via this route in intrapelvic metastases. Certainly for the bulky diseases, it can produce some rapid and dramatic responses.

Oncology 1993;50(suppl 1):53–62

Lawrence R. Coia

Fox Chase Cancer Center and University of Pennsylvania School of Medicine, Philadelphia, Pa., USA

The Use of Mitomycin in Esophageal Cancer

Key Words
Mitomycin
Esophageal cancer

Abstract
Concurrent administration of chemotherapeutic agents and radiation with or without surgery has yielded better local disease control and more prolonged survival than has standard radiation therapy or surgery alone in patients with esophageal cancer. Combinations of 5-fluorouracil (5-FU) and either cisplatin or mitomycin have proven most effective in this setting. As a single agent, mitomycin has generated response rates of 14–42% in patients with squamous cell carcinoma of the esophagus. The response of patients with esophageal adenocarcinoma to single-agent mitomycin is unknown. The clinical use of mitomycin concurrent with 5-FU and radiation is well established in esophageal cancer. There is some experimental evidence to suggest that synergy may occur between 5-FU and mitomycin. Mitomycin is preferentially cytotoxic to hypoxic cells, which are relatively radioresistant. It is not clear whether use of mitomycin with radiation is additive or supra-additive as experimental evidence exists to support both types of interaction. Nonrandomized clinical trials suggest that using either cisplatin or mitomycin concurrently with 5-FU and relatively low-dose radiation (30 Gy) prior to esophagectomy can result in comparable rates of pathologic complete response (20–30%) and median survival (12–19 months). Hematologic toxicity is frequently severe if all 3 drugs are used concurrently in combination with radiation. In patients with advanced disease (stage III or IV), combination chemotherapy/radiation therapy can result in significant palliation with tolerable morbidity. The use of concurrent chemotherapy and radiation has changed the pattern of failure in esophageal cancer from one dominated by inability to control local disease to one where systemic failure predominates. Current and proposed trials in esophageal cancer have changed their focus accordingly to meet this new treatment challenge.

Overall results obtained with standard use of radiation therapy or surgery alone in the treatment of esophageal cancer have been generally quite poor, with fewer than 10% of patients surviving 5 years [1]. Yet during the past decade promising new approaches to the clinical treatment of esophageal cancer have evolved. Pilot studies have suggested that the concurrent use of chemotherapy and radiation therapy with or without surgery may improve both local disease control and survival over standard therapies. Furthermore, recent data from phase III

Lawrence R. Coia, MD
Fox Chase Cancer Center
Radiation Oncology
Central & Shelmire Avenues
Philadelphia, PA 19111 (USA)

0030–2414/93/0507–0053
$2.75/0

trials of concurrent chemotherapy and radiation therapy versus radiation alone indicate improved results are obtained when concurrent therapy is used.

The purpose of this review is to evaluate the role of mitomycin in the treatment of esophageal cancer, with an emphasis on results of clinical trials employing concurrent radiation and chemotherapy with or without surgery. Although the predominant histologic subtype of esophageal cancer in the United States is squamous cell carcinoma, the incidence of adenocarcinoma is increasing [2]. Thus, the role of mitomycin in both subtypes will be reviewed.

Use of Mitomycin in Advanced Esophageal Cancer

Single-Agent Trials

Squamous Cell Carcinoma. Use of mitomycin as a single agent has proven effective in the treatment of advanced squamous cell carcinoma of the esophagus, with reported overall response rates of 14–42% [3–6]. Response rates in patients with locoregional cancer are usually higher than those seen in patients with advanced disease, and criteria for response evaluation often differ between studies. In early studies of mitomycin in squamous cell carcinoma of the esophagus, Cook and Bradner [3] reported a 15% subjective response rate while Desai et al. [4] observed a nearly 50% subjective response (14 of 27 patients) but an objective response of only 15% (4 patients). Whittington and Close [5] reported an objective response of only 14% (1 of 7 patients) using a dose schedule of 0.05 mg/kg/day mitomycin for 10 days.

The Eastern Cooperative Oncology Group (ECOG) examined the activity of mitomycin and that of cisplatin in a phase II trial in patients with advanced squamous cell carcinoma of the esophagus using standard ECOG criteria for toxicity and solid tumor response. Engstrom et al. [6] reported the results in 1983. Mitomycin was administered at a dose of 20 mg/m^2 i.v. every 4 weeks for two courses and every 6 weeks until evidence of disease progression or serious toxicity was noted. The mitomycin treatment program yielded a 42% partial response (PR) rate (10 of 24 patients), a median response duration of 12 weeks, and a median survival duration of 14 weeks. The cisplatin regimen produced a 25% PR rate (6 of 24 patients), a median response duration of 16 weeks, and a median survival duration of 18 weeks. Hematologic toxicity was higher in patients treated with mitomycin; 5 patients experienced severe myelosuppression and an additional 8 significant but less severe marrow depression. As Kelsen [7] pointed out in a review of the use of chemotherapy in esophageal cancer, mitomycin appears to induce one of the highest single-agent response rates, but this high response rate may be obtained at the cost of prohibitive toxicity.

Adenocarcinoma. Since adenocarcinoma of the esophagus occurs less frequently, results of its treatment with single-agent chemotherapy are usually combined with those obtained in the treatment of squamous cell cancer of the esophagus. Although the two subtypes are thought to behave clinically in a similar way, response rates to chemotherapy may differ markedly [8]. Extensive experience in the use of mitomycin in the treatment of advanced adenocarcinoma of the gastrointestinal tract has yielded objective response rates of 18–30% [9, 10]. Approximations of the response rates of patients with esophageal adenocarcinoma may be obtained from this experience. Moertel et al. [9] reported approximately an 18% objective response rate among patients with advanced gastrointestinal cancer, the great majority of whom had primary colon tumors. The mean duration of tumor regression was relatively short at only 3 months. Comis and Carter [10] reviewed the results of multiple trials using single-agent mitomycin in advanced gastric cancer. Sixty-three of a total of 211 patients responded to treatment, for an overall objective response rate of 30%. The authors indicated that an intermittent dose schedule could lead to more manageable levels of hematopoietic toxicity than the use of small doses over protracted treatment times.

Combination Chemotherapy

The use of mitomycin in combination with other chemotherapy in the treatment of advanced squamous cell carcinoma of the esophagus is largely unstudied. Its efficacy as part of multiagent chemotherapy for adenocarcinoma of the esophagus can only be estimated from the response rates that occur when mitomycin is combined with 5-fluorouracil (5-FU) in the treatment of patients with adenocarcinoma of the stomach.

Biologic Basis for Use of Mitomycin with 5-FU and Radiation

In vitro studies indicate that mitomycin is preferentially cytotoxic to chronically hypoxic cells, suggesting that the drug's cell killing effect when used with radiation is additive rather than synergistic [11]. However, Grau and Overgaard [12] have investigated the radiosensitizing and cytotoxic properties of mitomycin in vivo using regrowth delay and tumor control assays and, using isobologram

Table 1. Results of selected studies employing preoperative concurrent chemotherapy and radiation

Investigator	Ref.	Chemotherapy	Radiation dose, Gy	Resection rate, %	Postoperative mortality, %	Pathologic CR, %	Median survival, months
Franklin et al.	16	5-FU/mitomycin	30	79	26	26 (6/23)[1]	19
Leichman et al.	17	5-FU/cisplatin	30	71	27	27 (5/19)	18
SWOG	18	5-FU/cisplatin	30	49	11	25 (18/71)	12
RTOG	19	5-FU/cisplatin	30	71	4	30 (8/27)	13[2]

SWOG = Southwest Oncology Group.
[1] Number of esophageal specimens free of residual cancer divided by number of resections.
[2] Mean survival.

analysis, have found that delivery of mitomycin before radiation therapy results in a supra-additive response, whereas delivery after radiation has only an additive effect. They have also shown that a single dose of mitomycin (3 mg/kg) kills up to 97% of all hypoxic tumor cells [12]. The preferential cytotoxicity of mitomycin to hypoxic cells is of potential value since chronically hypoxic cells are relatively resistant to radiation and most chemotherapy. Work by Brown et al. [13] from Stanford indicates that use of a hypoxic cytotoxin with radiation can produce more tumor cell kill (by several orders of magnitude) than can either full oxygenation of a tumor or use of a 'perfect' hypoxic cell sensitizer under certain conditions. Such conditions exist, for example, provided that the hypoxic cytotoxin kills approximately 50% or more of the hypoxic cells each time it is given and that some reoxygenation occurs during delivery of the fractionated course of radiation [13].

An active single agent in patients with esophageal cancer, 5-FU may also act synergistically with radiation [14]. Clinically, mitomycin is frequently combined with 5-FU in the treatment of esophageal cancer and other gastrointestinal malignancies. Using isobologram analysis, Dobrowsky et al. [15] demonstrated in an in vitro model a greater than additive interaction between 5-FU and mitomycin. Therefore, the clinical effectiveness of regimens containing 5-FU/mitomycin/radiation in theory may derive in part from the potential synergy of 5-FU with mitomycin, of radiation with 5-FU, and of radiation with mitomycin.

Trials of Preoperative Chemotherapy and Radiation Therapy

The results of selected trials employing preoperative concurrent chemotherapy and radiation are shown in table 1 [16–19]. The first trial of concurrent chemotherapy and radiation therapy given preoperatively to patients with esophageal cancer was conducted by Franklin et al. [16] of Wayne State University. This group had developed and successfully used a regimen of 5-FU/mitomycin/radiation in patients with anal cancer and subsequently applied it to esophageal cancer. Thirty patients were treated with radiation (30 Gy, days 1–21) along with 5-FU (1,000 mg/m^2/day, days 1–4 and 29–32) and mitomycin (10 mg/m^2 day 1) followed by surgery (days 49–64). Postoperative chemotherapy plus an additional 20-Gy radiation was given to patients with residual cancer at surgery. Preoperative assessment included endoscopy with biopsy and an esophagogram.

Response to this regimen was excellent, with only 1 of 23 patients showing histologic evidence of disease at the presurgical endoscopic evaluation. Six of the 23 patients (26%) who underwent esophagectomy had no evidence of cancer in the resected specimen, and 3 others had only intraluminal tumor remaining. Further follow-up showed that no patient with residual tumor in the resected esophagus remained alive without disease, while 4 of the 6 patients without tumor in the resected specimen survived 95–190 weeks. One patient who refused surgery following radiation and infusional chemotherapy was alive at 4 years. The median survival in this group was 19 months. Postoperative mortality was high (26%) and was ascribed to high concentrations (>50%) of inspired oxygen in the postoperative period and possibly also to mitomycin use.

Following their successful use of cisplatin in advanced esophageal cancer, the Wayne State group modified the 5-FU/mitomycin protocol, substituting cisplatin (100 mg/m^2 days 1 and 29) for mitomycin [17]. Of 21 patients treated with the modified regimen, 19 underwent surgery, with 5 (27%) showing no cancer in the resected esophagus. Postoperative mortality, however, remained high, with 5 of 19 patients (27%) dying postoperatively. Median survival was 18 months for all patients and 24 months for those with no tumor in the resected specimen. Thus, nearly identical rates of response, survival, and toxicity were seen at the same institution, regardless of whether mitomycin or cisplatin was combined with 5-FU and radiation as part of the preoperative treatment regimen.

The regimen of 5-FU/cisplatin/radiation followed by esophagectomy was further studied in separate phase II trials conducted by the Southwest Oncology Group [18] and the Radiation Therapy Oncology Group (RTOG) [19]. Results were generally inferior to those reported in the initial Wayne State trials, as neither group obtained survival results that differed significantly from those obtainable with surgery alone or radiation alone. It is noteworthy that both cooperative group studies observed a higher median survival in responders compared with non-responders. In general, the only long-term survivors were those patients who had no evidence of tumor in the esophagectomy specimen.

Although 5-FU and mitomycin or cisplatin have frequently been combined with radiation in the treatment of esophageal cancer, only a few trials have used all 3 drugs in combination with radiation and subsequent surgery. At the University of Virginia, Stewart et al. [20] reported the results of a trial in which patients with esophageal cancer received all 3 agents concurrently with radiation therapy with or without esophagectomy. All 29 patients were treated with 5-FU (1,000 mg/m^2/day) continuous intravenous infusion days 1–4, cisplatin (100 mg/m^2) i.v. on day 1, and mitomycin (10 mg/m^2) i.v. on day 1. Significant hematologic toxicity was observed with this treatment regimen. Fever and neutropenia requiring broad-spectrum antibiotic therapy developed in 11 of 29 patients; however, all patients recovered without sequelae. Nine of 29 patients suffered grade 4 leukopenia. Surgical complications included respiratory failure requiring ventilatory support (3 patients). Overall, the hematologic toxicity of this regimen appears to be greater than that of regimens employing only 2 of these agents or non-concurrent use of these 3 agents.

Concurrent Chemotherapy/Radiation Therapy as Definitive Management of Esophageal Cancer

While others tested the use of concurrent radiation and infusional 5-FU with mitomycin or cisplatin preoperatively, several investigators examined the use of concurrent radiation and chemotherapy without surgery. At the Fox Chase Cancer Center, a pilot study begun in 1980 used conventional radiation therapy (to 60 Gy) with two 96-hour infusions of 5-FU (1 g/m^2, days 2–5 and 29–32) and a bolus intravenous injection of mitomycin (10 mg/m^2, day 2). Results obtained in 90 patients treated prospectively with this regimen, with a median follow-up time of 45 months, have been reported [21]. Fifty-seven patients with stage I or II disease received definitive radiation consisting of 60 Gy given over 6–7 weeks with the above chemotherapy, while 33 patients with stage III, IV, or otherwise advanced disease received palliative radiation treatment of 50 Gy over 5 weeks plus the same chemotherapy.

The overall median survival of patients with stage I or II disease was 18 months, with 3- and 5-year actuarial survivals of 29 and 18%, respectively. Median disease-specific survival was 20 months, with 3- and 5-year actuarial disease-specific survivals of 41 and 30%, respectively (fig. 1). A multivariate analysis of sex, histology, tumor location, and tumor size revealed that the effect of stage on survival was highly significant (stage I vs. stage II: 73 vs. 33% at 3 years, $p = 0.01$), whereas the effect of sex approached significance (females vs. males: 57 vs. 34% at 3 years, $p<0.1$). The actuarially determined local relapse-free rate for patients with stage I and II disease at both 3 and 5 years was 70%. Multivariate analysis also indicated stage had a significant impact on local tumor control (stage I vs. stage II: 100 vs. 60% at 3 years, $p<0.01$), whereas the effect of sex approached significance (females vs. males: 75 vs. 66% at 3 years, $p = 0.07$).

The median survival of patients with stage III or IV disease was 9 and 7 months, respectively. Palliation in this group was good, as 77% were rendered free of dysphagia posttreatment and 60% were without dysphagia until death, with a median dysphagia-free duration of 5 months. These results demonstrate that concurrent administration of 5-FU/mitomycin/radiation is an effective palliative treatment for patients with advanced esophageal cancer.

Severe toxicities were uncommon and nearly all were transient. Eleven of 90 patients (12.2%) had severe acute toxicities, while only 3 (3.3%) developed significant treatment-related complications requiring hospitalization. Persistent leukopenia precluded second courses of 5-FU

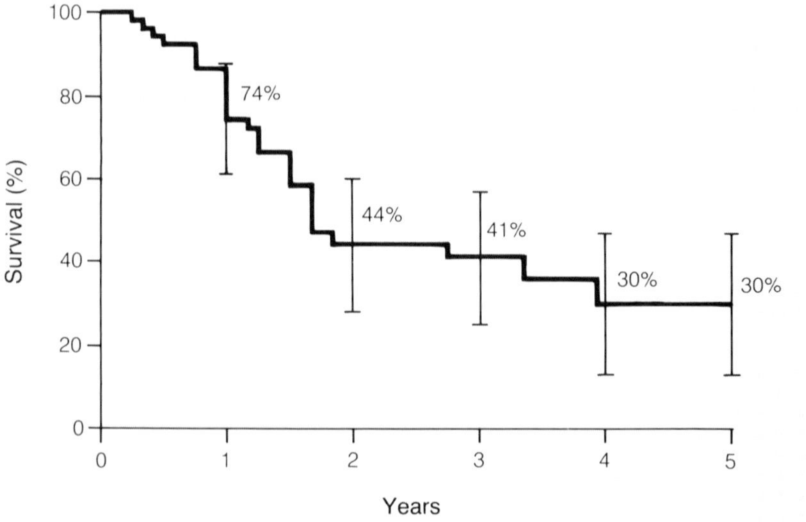

Fig. 1. Actuarial disease-specific survival of patients with stage I or II esophageal cancer. Twenty-seven of a total 57 patients died of their disease. Vertical solid lines = 95% confidence intervals. From Coia et al. [21], with permission.

in only 4 of 90 patients (4.4%), while 14 patients (15.5%) required a 25% dose reduction in the second course of 5-FU due to moderate hematologic depression. No patients had severe or life-threatening pancytopenia. One patient developed transient pneumonitis, and 1 patient died of complications related to the development of pneumonitis and later mediastinitis. The results of this study do not substantiate the concern expressed by some investigators regarding the pulmonary toxicity of radiation combined with mitomycin. The observed rate of pulmonary toxicity of only 2% (2 of 90 patients) is less than that reported in studies using radiation alone for esophageal cancer. Pulmonary toxicity is a function of the volume of lung that receives doses above those tolerable; thus careful attention to the technique of radiation delivery can minimize this complication, as was seen in this study. In particular, the use of a three-field technique (two posterior-oblique and an anterior field) throughout treatment delivers a higher dose to a larger volume of lung than does use of anterior and posterior fields for at least half of treatment followed by a three-field technique.

Table 2 [21–25] shows results of several studies that used definitive radiation and concurrent chemotherapy without surgery. Keane et al. [22] used infusional 5-FU and mitomycin along with either continuous single-course radiation to 50 Gy over 4 weeks or split-course radiation with a 4-week rest between treatments. Results suggested an improvement in local relapse-free survival among patients receiving single-course compared with split-course treatment; however, a bias in patient selection favored single-course treatment. Chan et al. [23] combined concurrent split-course radiation and infusional 5-FU with alternating administration of mitomycin/cisplatin in patients with advanced inoperable esophageal cancer and reported sustained palliation of dysphagia with acceptable morbidity. Leichman et al. [24] reported a median survival of 22 months using a 4-drug regimen of 5-FU/cisplatin/mitomycin/bleomycin with concurrent radiation therapy. Six patients were alive without cancer at 22–39 months. Observed clinical pulmonary toxicity was ascribed to bleomycin and mitomycin, for which the investigators later substituted additional courses of 5-FU/cisplatin. At present, at least four nonrandomized studies suggest improved survival in patients treated with concurrent radiation and chemotherapy compared with matched historical controls who received radiation alone [22, 23, 25, 26].

These studies suggest regimens of concurrent radiation and chemotherapy may alter the treatment failure pattern from one of local failure to one dominated by distant metastases. The report of Coia et al. [21] showed that, of 29 patients who developed recurrent disease, 14 (48%) had some component of local failure whereas 21 (72%) had a component of distant failure. Likewise, Chan et al. [23] compared the failure patterns of 21 patients treated with split-course radiation and concurrent infusional 5-FU and mitomycin to those of 34 patients treated with radiation alone. In the radiation and chemotherapy group, 47% had a component of local failure and 71% a component of distant failure.

Table 2. Results of selected studies employing concurrent radiation and chemotherapy with mitomycin

Investigator	Ref.	Patients, n	Chemotherapy	Radiation dose, Gy	1-year local relapse-free survival, %	Median survival, months	Survival at 2 years, %	Survival at 5 years, %	Treatment-related mortality, %
Keane et al.	22	15	Mitomycin/5-FU	45–50	79		48	–	0
		20		22.5–25 × 2 (split course)	27	12	12	–	0
Chan et al.	23	21	Mitomycin/5-FU	20–25 × 2 (split course)	67	13	32	–	0
Leichman et al.	24	20	Mitomycin/5-FU/ bleomycin/ cisplatin	50 (split course)	60	22	35	–	5 (1/20) UGI hemorrhage
John et al.	25	30	Mitomycin/5-FU/ cisplatin plus maintenance therapy (methotrexate/ 5-FU/leucovorin)	41.4–50.4	73	11	29	–	3 (1/30) pulmonary fibrosis
Coia et al.	21								
Stage I, II		57	Mitomycin/5-FU	60	75	18[1]	34[1]	18	2 (2/90) Mediastinitis (MI)
Stage III, IV		33		50	60[2]	8			

UGI = Upper gastrointestinal; MI = myocardial infarction.

[1] Disease-specific survival; overall survival at 2 and 5 years is 34 and 18%, respectively.

[2] Measured as sustained palliation rather than local relapse-free survival.

Two randomized cooperative group studies have examined concurrent radiation and chemotherapy versus radiation alone in patients with esophageal cancer. An ECOG trial compared radiation alone (to 60 Gy) with radiation (to 60 Gy) plus concurrent infusional 5-FU and mitomycin, with an option for surgical resection after 40 Gy, in patients with distal lesions. Preliminary analysis indicates that median survival in the group receiving concurrent radiation and chemotherapy is 14.9 versus 9 months in the group receiving radiation therapy alone ($p = 0.03$) [27]. In a trial initiated by the RTOG, cisplatin (75 mg/m^2) and 5-FU (1,000 mg/m^2/day × 4 days) given in two concurrent courses with radiation (to 50 Gy) followed by two courses of the same chemotherapy was compared with radiation alone (to 64 Gy). Again, the interim results favor concurrent treatment with radiation/chemotherapy. Two-year survival in the bimodality arm was 42 versus 10% in the radiation alone arm ($p = 0.0017$) [28]. The results of these trials indicate that radiation therapy alone can no longer be considered a standard therapy for patients with esophageal cancer.

Future Studies

Having made some progress in local disease control and survival in the treatment of esophageal cancer, clinical oncologists have begun to focus on the problem of distant metastases. At present, chemotherapy trials proposed or in progress are, in general, focusing on neoadjuvant use of cisplatin/5-FU combinations that have attained objective response rates of about 50% in patients with advanced esophageal cancer.

In the treatment of adenocarcinoma of the esophagus, Coia et al. [21, 29] have shown that radiation and concurrent chemotherapy can provide significant local tumor control, palliation, and the chance for long-term survival in patients with inoperable or unresectable disease or in patients who refuse surgery. Surgery, however, remains the mainstay of treatment in patients with resectable adenocarcinoma of the esophagus. Whittington et al. [30], in a retrospective review of a variety of therapeutic approaches to esophageal adenocarcinoma, suggest that trimodality treatment, i.e., concurrent radiation and chemotherapy given preoperatively or postoperatively, offers improved results over other treatment strategies. ECOG is presently performing a pilot study in patients with adenocarcinoma of the esophagus, using the Fox Chase regimen of concurrent radiation (60 Gy) and chemotherapy with 5-FU/mitomycin followed by esophageal resection.

Conclusion

Clinical studies using mitomycin as a component of concurrent chemotherapy and radiation in the treatment of esophageal cancer have provided excellent results with tolerable toxicity. Regimens of concurrent radiation plus chemotherapy represent preferred alternatives to esophagectomy or radiation alone in the primary management of squamous cell carcinoma of the esophagus and are an effective treatment for patients with adenocarcinoma of the esophagus as well. Two properties of mitomycin may make it particularly useful when combined with radiation therapy: its preferential cytotoxicity to hypoxic cells and its potential synergy with 5-FU. Results of trials using infusional 5-FU, mitomycin, and concurrent radiation are comparable with those of trials using regimens in which cisplatin is substituted for mitomycin. The possibility of conducting a randomized study examining 5-FU/mitomycin/concurrent radiation versus 5-FU/cisplatin/concurrent radiation is currently being explored. Subgroups of patients may exist that are better treated with regimens containing mitomycin than cisplatin (e.g., patients with adenocarcinoma or patients with tumors containing large hypoxic fractions). Acute toxicity, particularly nausea and emesis, occurs less frequently with mitomycin than with cisplatin. Only a well-designed phase III trial comparing these two different chemotherapeutic components of a successful concurrent radiation/chemotherapy regimen can determine their relative efficacy and toxicity.

Acknowledgments

The author wishes to thank Dr. Seth Rosenthal for his helpful comments and Louise Marcewicz for her skillful preparation of the manuscript.

References

1 Earlam R, Cunha-Melo JR: Esophageal squamous cell carcinoma: A critical review of radiotherapy. Br J Surg 1980;67:457–461.
2 Hesketh PJ, Clapp RW, Doos WG, et al: The increasing frequency of adenocarcinoma of the esophagus. Cancer 1980;64:526–530.
3 Cook ST, Bradner WT: Mitomycin C-A review. Cancer Treat Rev 1976;3:121–139.
4 Desai P, Borges E, Vohrs V, et al: Carcinoma of the esophagus in India. Cancer 1969;23:979–989.
5 Whittington R, Close H: Clinical experiences with mitomycin C. Cancer Chemother Rep 1970;54:195–198.
6 Engstrom P, Lavin P, Kallsen D: Phase II evaluation of mitomycin and cisplatin in advanced esophageal carcinoma. Cancer Treat Rep 1983;67:713–715.
7 Kelsen D: Chemotherapy for local-regional and advanced esophageal cancer. Cancer Updates 1988;2(10):1–12.
8 Forastiere A, Gevnis M, Orringer M, et al: A trial of cisplatin, vinblastine and mitoguazone chemotherapy for epidermoid and adenocarcinoma of the esophagus. J Clin Oncol 1987;5:1143–1149.
9 Moertel CG, Reitemeier RJ, Hahn RG: Mitomycin C therapy in advanced gastrointestinal cancer. JAMA 1968;204:111–114.
10 Comis RL, Carter SK: A review of chemotherapy in gastric cancer. Cancer 1974;34:1576–1586.
11 Rockwell S, Kennedy K: Combination therapy with radiation and mitomycin-C: Preliminary results with EMT-6 tumor cells in vitro and in vivo. Int J Radiat Oncol Biol Phys 1979;5:1673–1676.
12 Grau C, Overgaard J: Radiosensitizing and cytotoxic properties of mitomycin C in a C3H mouse mammary carcinoma in vivo. Int J Radiat Oncol Biol Phys 1991;20:265–269.
13 Brown JM, Koong A, Lemmon M: A comparison of the relative efficacies of combining either a hypoxic cell radiosensitizer, increased tumor oxygenation or a hypoxic cytotoxin with fractionated irradiation (abstract). 7th Int Conf Chem Modif Cancer Treat, Clearwater, Fla., 1991, pp 272–273.
14 Byfield JE, Calabro-Jones P, Klisak I, et al: Pharmacologic requirements for obtaining sensitization of human tumor cells in vitro to combined 5-fluorouracide or ftorafur and x-rays. Int J Radiat Oncol Biol Phys 1982;8:1923–1933.
15 Dobrowsky W, Dobrowsky E, Rauth AM: Mode of interaction of 5-fluorouracil (5-FU), radiation, and mitomycin C (MMC): In vitro studies (abstr). 3rd Int Conf Interaction Radiat Ther Systemic Ther. Monterey, March 1990, p 1–2A – 1–2C.
16 Franklin R, Steiger Z, Vaishampayan G, et al: Combined modality therapy for esophageal squamous cell carcinoma. Cancer 1983;51:1062–1071.
17 Leichman L, Steiger Z, Seydel HG, et al: Preoperative chemotherapy and radiation therapy for patients with cancer of the esophagus: A potentially curative approach. J Clin Oncol 1984;2:75–79.
18 Poplin E, Fleming T, Leichman L, et al: Combined therapies for squamous cell carcinoma of the esophagus, a Southwest Oncology Group Study (SWOG-8037). J Clin Oncol 1987;5:622–628.
19 Seydel HG, Leichman L, Byhardt R, et al: Preoperative radiation and chemotherapy for localized squamous cell carcinoma of the esophagus: A RTOG study. Int J Radiat Oncol Biol Phys 1988;14:33–35.

20 Stewart FM, Harkins J, Hahn SS, et al: Cisplatin, 5-fluorouracil, mitomycin C and concurrent radiation therapy with and without esophagectomy for esophageal carcinoma. Cancer 1989;64:622–628.

21 Coia LR, Engstrom PF, Paul AR, et al: Long-term results of infusional 5-FU, mitomycin C and radiation as primary management of esophageal carcinoma. Int J Radiat Oncol Biol Phys 1991;20:29–37.

22 Keane TJ, Harwood AR, Elhakim T, et al: Radical radiation therapy with 5-fluorouracil infusion and mitomycin C for oesophageal squamous carcinoma. Radiother Oncol 1985; 4:205–210.

23 Chan A, Wong A, Arthur K: Concomitant 5-FU infusion, mitomycin-C and radical therapy in esophageal squamous cell carcinoma. Int J Radiat Oncol Biol Phys 1989;16:59–65.

24 Leichman L, Herskovic A, Leichman CG, et al: Nonoperative therapy for squamous cell cancer of the esophagus. J Clin Oncol 1987;5: 365–370.

25 John M, Flam M, Ager Mowry P, et al: Radiotherapy alone and chemoradiation for non-metastatic esophageal carcinoma. Cancer 1989;63:2397–2403.

26 Richmond J, Seydel HG, Bae Y, et al: Comparison of three treatment strategies for esophageal cancer within a single institution. Int J Radiat Oncol Biol Phys 1987;13:1617–1620.

27 Sischy B, Ryan L, Haller D, et al: Interim report of EST 1282: A phase III protocol for the evaluation of combined modalities in the treatment of patients with carcinoma of the esophagus, stage I & II (abstract). Proc Am Soc Clin Oncol 1990;9:105.

28 Herskovic A, Martz K, Al-Sarraf M, et al: Intergroup Esophageal Study: Comparison of radiotherapy (RT) to radio-chemotherapy combination. A phase III trial (abstract). Proc Am Soc Clin Oncol 1991;10:135.

29 Coia L, Paul A, Engstrom P: Combined radiation and chemotherapy as primary management of adenocarcinoma of the esophagus and gastro-esophageal junction. Cancer 1988;61: 643–649.

30 Whittington R, Coia L, Haller D, et al: Adenocarcinoma of the esophagus and esophagogastric junction: The effects of single and combined modalities on the survival and patterns of failure following treatment. Int J Radiat Oncol Biol Phys 1990;19:593–603.

Discussion

Dr. Henderson: Dr. Coia, based on the data that you presented and the studies that you have illustrated, what do you see as the current role for surgery in patients with esophageal tumors?

Dr. Coia: At Fox Chase Cancer Center, the regimen that we have used (and that has been used elsewhere), namely, concurrent mitomycin, 5-fluorouracil (5-FU), and radiation, is relatively effective in the treatment of patients with squamous cell cancer of the esophagus. There may not be a role for surgery unless we identify particular subgroups of patients whose tumors are not responsive to concurrent radiation and chemotherapy.

At present, we feel there is a role for surgery in the patient with esophageal adenocarcinoma. For example, some of the best results reported in esophageal cancer came from the University of Michigan, and were reported in the *Journal of Clinical Oncology* last year by Arlene Forestiere. The regimen used included cisplatin, vinblastine, and 5-FU with concurrent hyperfractionated radiotherapy followed by transhiatal esophagectomy. Approximately half of the patients had adenocarcinoma and half had squamous cell cancer. The 3-year survival of patients with adenocarcinoma was 56%. These results are quite promising, but it must be realized that follow-up was relatively short (26 months) and there were only 21 patients with adenocarcinoma. We are currently conducting a pilot study of 5-FU, mitomycin, and high-dose radiation (60 Gy), followed by esophagectomy in patients with adenocarcinoma. Unfortunately, there has never been a randomized trial comparing concurrent radiation and chemotherapy versus surgery for esophageal cancer. It is very difficult to conduct that type of a trial in the United States.

Dr. Keane: One major four-arm randomized trial in Hong Kong compared surgery, radiotherapy, preoperative radiotherapy and surgery, and surgery and postoperative radiotherapy in patients with squamous carcinoma. I understand from discussions with Dr. J. Wong (personal communication) that there was no difference in survival between any of the arms. So, I think it has already been established in at least one trial – and certainly in the historical literature – that there is no difference between radiotherapy and surgery with regard to long-term survival results.

The argument has always been about palliation – whether patients having radiotherapy can swallow as well as patients having surgery. In the United States, surgery has dominated the treatment of cancer of the esophagus and certainly squamous carcinoma. In many centers in Canada, radiotherapy has for a long time been more or less the definitive treatment for lesions at or above the level of the carina of the trachea. And I think results of studies performed there give further impetus to a much stronger nonsurgical approach.

I think the key issue, though, is to come back to what we are here to discuss – why mitomycin is the active agent of choice for the treatment of esophageal tumors. Having treated over 200 patients with either mitomycin/5-FU or 5-FU alone, we find that the trend in our data strongly indicates that you cannot afford to leave mitomycin out of the regimen.

Dr. Coia: Our medical oncologists feel the mitomycin/5-FU-based regimen is quite tolerable and probably more tolerable than cisplatin-based regimens. With regard to why neoadjuvant chemotherapy is being looked at now, as I pointed out, the predominant pattern of failure is no longer local but, rather, distant. We are attempting to improve survival by decreasing the systemic tumor burden by the use of intensified up-front chemotherapy.

Question: How many courses of concomitant therapy and how many courses of chemotherapy after completion of radiotherapy do patients receive?

Dr. Coia: In our trial patients received concomitant chemotherapy and radiation therapy for only 2 weeks and no additional chemotherapy after completion of concurrent therapy. More recently we have piloted the use of additional monthly 5-FU after concurrent radiation and chemotherapy, but patients have found this difficult to tolerate. In their randomized trial, the Eastern Cooperative Oncology Group (ECOG) employed exactly the same chemotherapy/radiation schedule as our initial large trial, i.e., without giving additional chemotherapy. The recent Radiation Therapy Oncology Group (RTOG) trial, however, included two additional cycles of cisplatin/5-FU following completion of concurrent chemotherapy/radiation.

Dr. Henderson: That is relatively short-duration therapy, which makes the results seem all the more impressive.

Dr. Schnall: I think there is reason, on theoretical grounds, to believe that using simultaneous chemoradiotherapy as neoadjuvant therapy might be a good way to go. There is likely to be synergism between the two approaches. The more you reduce tumor bulk with preoperative preradiotherapy chemotherapy, the greater your chances may be of getting a better result. So that approach might be worth exploring.

Dr. Coia: We are currently proposing a trial of intensive cisplatin neoadjuvant chemotherapy, but we have no intention of reducing the dose of radiation in the subsequent delivery of concurrent radiation and chemotherapy.

Dr. Henderson: You might not want to do that immediately. But, if you find that your incidence of pathologically confirmed or complete remissions is very high, you might want to reduce the dose at some future time.

Dr. Coia: Yes, possibly.

Dr. Keane: I was very upset to see that the RTOG had dropped the dose of radiation in the radiation and chemotherapy arm, and were comparing it with 64 Gy in their trial of radiotherapy with and without cisplatin and 5-FU. We have consistently used doses equivalent to about 60 or 62 Gy with the same mitomycin regimen without any difficulty. Reduction of the radiation dose could compromise what otherwise might be an effective chemoradiotherapy regimen. I think people have to be very concerned about dose reduction that might negate the value of a new and promising treatment.

Dr. Coia: There are also some potential problems with neoadjuvant treatment. For example, the existence of accelerated tumor repopulation during treatment and the various stimuli that may provoke it have raised a serious concern in the radiotherapy community. Namely, does neoadjuvant chemotherapy result in accelerated repopulation prior to and during radiation? Why, for instance, in cancer of the nasopharynx, a remarkably chemosensitive disease, has neoadjuvant chemotherapy failed to have an impact despite achieving initial response rates of up to 80%. One possible explanation is that, despite the high responses with neoadjuvant chemotherapy, the tumor cell population is proliferating more rapidly by the time radiotherapy starts. This is a potentially serious problem of neoadjuvant studies.

Dr. Folman: Dr. Coia, do you feel that the administration of chemotherapy concurrently with radiation increases the severity of esophagitis compared with radiotherapy alone?

Dr. Coia: I cannot answer from our trial whether severity of esophagitis is increased, but I think it will be very interesting to analyze the results of the RTOG and ECOG trials in this regard. My personal opinion is yes, there probably is a slight increase in the severity of acute (not late) esophagitis with 5-FU/mitomycin, and perhaps even more so with 5-FU/cisplatin. But in only a few patients has esophagitis been severe enough to necessitate prolonged interruption of treatment or hospitalization for management.

Question: Have any of the delayed or unusual toxicities associated with mitomycin use in patients with breast cancer – hemolytic, uremic, or pulmonary – been observed in patients with esophageal cancer?

Dr. Coia: I have not seen any.

Oncology 1993;50(suppl 1):63–69

Bernard J. Cummings
Thomas J. Keane
Brian O'Sullivan
C. Shun Wong
Charles N. Catton

Department of Radiation Oncology,
The Princess Margaret Hospital,
Toronto, Ont., Canada

Mitomycin in Anal Canal Carcinoma

Key Words
Anal canal cancer
Mitomycin
5-Fluorouracil
Radiation therapy

Abstract
One hundred and ten patients with primary epidermoid cancers of the anal canal were treated in a series of prospectively designed, nonrandomized protocols of split-course radiation therapy with concurrent administration of 5-fluorouracil (5-FU) with or without mitomycin. The addition of mitomycin was associated with improved primary tumor control rates (87 vs. 58% at 4 years, $p = 0.005$) and improved 4-year actuarial cause-specific survival (80 vs. 64%, $p = 0.02$). Hematologic toxicity was the most frequent acute side effect of mitomycin use. No long-term toxicity was attributed to mitomycin only. Mitomycin appeared to benefit patients principally through improved control of cancer in the irradiated volume; there was no evidence of reduced risk of extrapelvic metastases. Several investigators have reported high rates of control of epidermoid anal cancers with preservation of anorectal function following concurrent treatment with mitomycin, 5-FU, and radiation. Mitomycin's role in anal cancer is being evaluated in a randomized clinical trial by the Radiation Therapy Oncology Group. The mechanisms of any interactions between mitomycin and radiation or other cytotoxic drugs in clinical practice remain to be determined.

Concurrent radiation therapy, mitomycin, and 5-fluorouracil (5-FU) are widely used to treat epidermoid carcinomas of the anal canal. This approach was introduced in 1972 at Wayne State University, where Nigro et al. [1] had observed responses to 5-FU and mitomycin given alone and in combination in small numbers of patients with metastatic anal cancers. Both drugs were then given in combination with radiation as adjuvant treatment prior to abdominoperineal resection, the then standard surgical procedure for most anal canal carcinomas. As it became clear that patients so treated frequently showed no residual cancer in tissue subsequently removed at surgery, the regimen gained increasing acceptance. Radical surgery requiring sacrifice of anorectal function was reserved for patients with residual cancer following radiation and chemotherapy or without anal competence.

The combination of radiation therapy, 5-FU, and mitomycin proved to be more effective for epidermoid cancers than for adenocarcinomas. Epidermoid cancers of the anal canal include squamous cell, basaloid (sometimes called cloacogenic), and the rare mucoepidermoid and undifferentiated tumors [2]. Squamous cell and basaloid cancers in particular respond similarly to radiation and chemotherapy and are generally not separated in the presentation of results. The anal canal is the terminal portion of the intestinal tract between the anal verge and the pal-

B.J. Cummings, MB
Department of Radiation Oncology
The Princess Margaret Hospital
500 Sherbourne Street
Toronto, Ont. M4X 1K9 (Canada)

0030–2414/93/0507–0063
$2.75/0

Table 1. Radiation/5-FU/mitomycin protocols (Princess Margaret Hospital)

Protocol	5-FU	Mitomycin	Radiation
1	1,000 mg/m^2/24 h 96-hour continuous i.v. infusion days 1–4 and 43–46	10 mg/m^2 i.v. bolus days 1 and 43	25 Gy/10 fractions days 1–12 and 43–54
2	1,000 mg/m^2/24 h 96-hour continuous i.v. infusion days 1–4 and 43–46	10 mg/m^2 i.v. bolus days 1 and 43	24 Gy/12 fractions days 1–16 and 43–59
3	1,000 mg/m^2/24 h 96-hour continuous i.v. infusion days 1–4 and 43–46		24 Gy/12 fractions days 1–16 and 43–59
4	1,000 mg/m^2/24 h 96-hour continuous i.v. infusion days 1–4 and 43–46		25 Gy/10 fractions days 1–12 and 43–54

pable upper border of the anal sphincters and puborectalis muscle of the anorectal ring [3]. The treatment of perianal skin cancers is not considered in this review.

The precise role of mitomycin in the combined-modality treatment of anal canal cancers is not known. At the Princess Margaret Hospital, however, a series of protocols for the management of anal cancers was developed sequentially and modified according to experience, especially with regard to acute normal tissue toxicity and primary tumor control rates. These studies suggest that mitomycin is an important element in the combination of mitomycin, 5-FU, and radiation [4]. The Radiation Therapy Oncology Group (RTOG) is conducting a trial in which patients are randomized to receive either 5-FU plus mitomycin or 5-FU alone concomitantly with radiation, and this trial should further clarify mitomycin's role.

The Princess Margaret Hospital Experience

Between 1981 and 1989, the Princess Margaret Hospital launched a series of four protocols designed to allow evaluation of mitomycin in combination with 5-FU and radiation therapy. A previous study had revealed that the combination of mitomycin, 5-FU, and uninterrupted radical radiation (50 Gy given in 20 fractions over 4 weeks) was effective but unduly toxic [5]. In the four protocols detailed here, patients received split-course radiation with concurrent short-course infusions of 5-FU; mitomycin was also given in two of these protocols (table 1) [4]. In the first protocol, split-course radiation was used to reduce the acute toxicity observed with uninterrupted irradiation and chemotherapy. This schedule was then modified by decreasing the daily fraction from 2.5 to 2 Gy in an effort to lessen further the severity of the acute perineal reaction. Because of concern over observed hematologic toxicity and the uncertain role of mitomycin in the program, mitomycin was deleted from the third and fourth protocols, which explored the effectiveness of split-course radiation (2 or 2.5 Gy/day) in combination with 5-FU alone.

Radiation therapy was given by megavoltage equipment. Interstitial brachytherapy was not used. Radiation was administered in split courses of either 25 Gy in 10 fractions over 2 weeks, separated by a 4-week split, or 24 Gy in 12 fractions over 2.5 weeks, separated by a 3.5-week split. The first half of treatment was delivered through anterior and posterior fields, which encompassed the primary tumor and iliac and inguinal nodes below the level of the lower end of the sacroiliac joints, with the dose prescribed at midplane. The second part was directed to a reduced volume that included the primary tumor only. Multiple-field arrangements were used most frequently, with the dose prescribed at the isocenter. Occasionally, treatment was given by a direct ^{60}Co perineal field, in which case the dose was prescribed at a depth of 3 cm. When histologically confirmed inguinal node metastases were present, anterior and posterior radiation fields were used for both the first and second treatment phases.

Chemotherapy consisted of a single bolus intravenous injection of mitomycin 10 mg/m^2 on the first day of each part of split-course radiation, without restriction of the

Table 2. Pretreatment patient characteristics

	Patients, n	
	5-FU/mitomycin/RT (n = 47)	5-FU/RT (n = 63)
Female: male ratio	30:17, or 1.8	34:29, or 1.2
Age range, years	32–87	30–88
Squamous cell carcinoma	37 (79)	42 (67)
Basaloid carcinoma	8 (17)	18 (29)
Other histology	2 (4)	3 (5)
UICC stage		
T_1 (≤2 cm)	7 (15)	9 (14)
T_2 (2.1–5 cm)	20 (43)	25 (40)
T_3 (>5 cm)	11 (23)	17 (27)
T_4 (invading adjacent organ)	9 (19)	11 (17)
N1–3	5 (11)	15 (24)

RT = Radiation therapy, UICC = International Union against Cancer.

Values in parentheses are percentages.

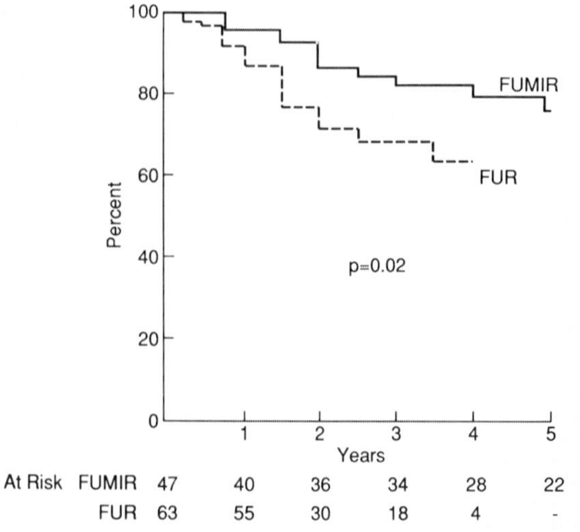

Fig. 1. Actuarial 4-year cause-specific survival among patients treated with 5-FU/mitomycin/radiation (FUMIR) or 5-FU/radiation (FUR).

maximum dose. 5-FU was given at 1,000 mg/m^2/24 h to a maximum of 1,500 mg/m^2/24 h by continuous peripheral i.v. infusion over the first 96 h of each course of radiation. Biopsies of the anal area were not routinely performed after irradiation and chemotherapy, except when residual tumor was suspected on clinical examination. When feasible, patients with residual cancer underwent attempted salvage surgery, usually abdominoperineal resection.

Forty-seven patients were treated with combined 5-FU, mitomycin, and radiation, and 63 with combined 5-FU and radiation. There were no major between-group differences in patient characteristics such as female-to-male ratios, histologic cancer types, or primary cancer T stages, but more patients treated with 5-FU and radiation had regional node metastases at presentation: 15/63 (24%) versus 5/47 (11%) (table 2) [4]. Actuarial 4-year, cause-specific survival rates were 80 and 64% for patients in the 5-FU/mitomycin/radiation and 5-FU/radiation groups, respectively ($p = 0.02$) (fig. 1). Survival rates by T stage did not differ significantly between the two treatment groups. Survival was not significantly affected by the presence at first treatment of clinically detectable, regional lymph node metastases.

Four-year primary tumor control rates were 87 and 58% for patients in the mitomycin- and nonmitomycin-containing arms, respectively ($p = 0.005$). Control rates according to primary tumor stage are shown in table 3 [4]. The mitomycin-containing protocols demonstrated an advantage for all tumor sizes greater than 2 cm. Overall primary tumor control rates were not influenced by the dose of radiation delivered each day (2 or 2.5 Gy). Residual primary cancers were controlled by surgery in 2 of 4 patients previously treated with 5-FU/mitomycin/radiation and in 5 of 17 previously treated with 5-FU/radiation. Anorectal function was preserved in 77 and 58% of patients following treatment with the mitomycin- and nonmitomycin-containing regimens, respectively. Continence was lost due to treatment-related toxicity in 3 and 2 patients treated with these regimens, respectively. Control of regional lymph node metastases identified at the time of first presentation occurred in 4 of 5 patients in the mitomycin-containing arm and in all 15 in the nonmitomycin-containing arm.

The mitomycin and nonmitomycin-containing arms failed to control pelvic cancer in either the primary site or regional lymph nodes within the irradiated volume in 8 of 47 (17%) and 27 of 62 (44%) patients, respectively; failure was confined to the pelvis in 5 (11%) and 22 (35%) of these patients. Extrapelvic metastases occurred either alone or in association with pelvic recurrence in 8 of 47 (17%) and 6 of 62 (10%) patients, respectively; such metastases represented the sole area of failure in 5 (11%) and 1 (2%) of these patients.

Table 3. Primary tumor control

	Number of complete responders/ total number of patients	
	5-FU/mitomycin/RT	5-FU/RT
UICC stage		
T_1 (≤2 cm)	7/7 (100)	8/9 (89)
T_2 (2.1–5 cm)	18/20 (90)	13/25 (52)
T_3 (>5 cm)	10/11 (91)	11/17 (65)
T_4 (invading adjacent organ)	6/9 (67)	4/11 (36)
Total	41/47 (87)	36/62[1] (58)

RT = Radiation therapy, UICC = International Union against Cancer.

Values in parentheses are percentages.

Adapted from Cummings et al [4].

[1] One patient died during treatment and so was not evaluable.

Table 6. Late toxicity (≥RTOG grade 3)

Radiation dose	Number of cases/total number of patients		
	5-FU/RT	5-FU/mitomycin/RT	Total (by radiation dose)
2 × 24 Gy	1/28	1/33	2/61 (3)*
2 × 25 Gy	5/34	5/14	10/48 (21)*
Total (by treatment)	6/62 (10)+	6/47 (13)+	

* $p = 0.004$; + $p = 0.62$.

RT = Radiation therapy.

Values in parentheses are percentages.

Table 4. Acute hematologic toxicity (≥RTOG grade 3)

Radiation dose	Number of cases/total number of patients		
	5-FU/RT	5-FU/mitomycin/RT	Total (by radiation dose)
2 × 24 Gy	1/29	9/33	10/62 (16)*
2 × 25 Gy	4/34	4/14	8/48 (17)*
Total (by treatment)	5/63 (8)+	13/47 (28)+	

* $p = 0.90$; + $p = 0.006$.

RT = Radiation therapy.

Values in parentheses are percentages.

Table 5. Acute nonhematologic toxicity (≥RTOG grade 3)

Radiation dose	Number of cases/total number of patients		
	5-FU/RT	5-FU/mitomycin/RT	Total (by radiation dose)
2 × 24 Gy	4/29	5/33	9/62 (15)*
2 × 25 Gy	5/34	5/14	10/48 (21)*
Total (by treatment)	9/63 (14)+	10/47 (21)+	

* $p = 0.39$; + $p = 0.34$.

RT = Radiation therapy.

Values in parentheses are percentages.

Incidence of severe (≥RTOG grade 3) hematologic and nonhematologic toxicity appears in tables 4 and 5. The dose of radiation administered each day (2 or 2.5 Gy) did not greatly affect the likelihood of severe acute toxicity in either treatment arm. Hematologic toxicity predominated among patients receiving the mitomycin-containing regimen. A hemoglobin decrease of 30 g/l or more occurred most frequently (10 of 47 patients, 21%); 2 patients had a nadir WBC count of less than 1×10^9/l, and 3 had a nadir platelet count of less than 50×10^9/l. There was no fatal toxicity, and no long-term toxicity attributable to mitomycin. One patient receiving 5-FU/radiation died during treatment of pneumonia without evidence of leukopenia.

The risk of serious late morbidity was lower in patients treated with 2 Gy/day radiation to a total of 48 Gy than in those treated with 2.5 Gy/day to a total of 50 Gy. The inclusion or omission of mitomycin did not appear to influence the risk of late toxicity in the split-course radiation schedules (table 6).

Recursive partition analysis [6] showed that the inclusion of mitomycin with radiation and 5-FU was the strongest predictor for local tumor control [4]. After review of the clinical significance of the hematologic toxicity observed, together with review of the toxicity reported by others who had used protocols combining mitomycin with radiation and 5-FU [7, 8], mitomycin has been reintroduced to the current Princess Margaret Hospital protocol for anal cancer.

Table 7. Selected trials of concurrent mitomycin/5-FU/radiation: results

Investigator	Ref.	Mitomycin[1]	5-FU[2]	Radiation (dose/fractions)	CRs/total patients		Survival, %
					n	%	
Nigro et al.	1	15 mg/m^2 day 1	1,000 mg/m^2/24 h days 1–4 and 29–32	30 Gy/15, days 1–20	97/104	93	5-year crude (80)
Sischy et al.	11	10 mg/m^2 day 2	1,000 mg/m^2/24 h days 2–5 and 28–31	40.8 Gy/24, days 1–35	57/65	88[3]	3-year actuarial (73)
Flam et al.	7	15 mg/m^2 days 1 and 30	1,000 mg/m^2/24 h days 1–4 and 30–34	41–45 Gy/25, days 1–35	27/30	90	27 NED 9–76 months
Papillon and Montbarbon	9	12 mg/m^2 day 1	600 mg/m^2/24 h days 1–5	42 Gy/10, days 1–16 plus interstitial 20 Gy day 77	57/70	81	Not stated
Cummings et al.	5	10 mg/m^2 day 1	1,000 mg/m^2/24 h days 1–4	50 Gy/20, days 1–26	14/16	88	5-year actuarial (75)
Cummings (present study)		10 mg/m^2 day 1 and approx. day 43	1,000 mg/m^2/24 h days 1–4 and approx. 43–46	48–50 Gy/24–20, split course, approx. days 1–58	41/47	87	5-year actuarial (65)

CRs = Complete responders; NED = no evidence of disease.
1 By i.v. bolus injection.
2 By continuous i.v. infusion.
3 Histologic complete regression rate.

Literature Review and Discussion

There have been no reports of the use of mitomycin as a single agent either alone or in combination with radiation for the treatment of primary anal carcinomas. However, an extensive body of data addresses the use of combined 5-FU and mitomycin, either concurrently with or sequentially to radiation. Data from nonrandomized comparisons suggest that for all tumors larger than 2 cm, local control rates with mitomycin, 5-FU, and radiation are superior to those achieved with radiation alone [4, 9]. It is hoped that randomized trials in progress in Europe and the United Kingdom will resolve whether the combination therapy is to be preferred to radiation alone.

The original protocol in which low-dose preoperative adjuvant radiation was combined with concurrent 5-FU and mitomycin [10] has been modified by several investigators, particularly by increases in the dose of radiation as the emphasis shifted from surgical adjuvant therapy to definitive treatment. Representative trials are shown in table 7 [1, 5, 7, 9, 11]. Despite differences in the doses of radiation and drugs used, and in the sizes of the tumors treated, about 80–90% of primary tumors have been controlled, and 5-year survival rates range from about 65–80%. While these survival rates are somewhat better than those reported in large series of patients treated with radiation alone, several studies with 5-FU, mitomycin, and radiation excluded patients with regional lymph node metastases, and whether the improvement in survival rates is real or reflects patient selection must await the outcome of randomized trials. The results obtained in our study show that regional node metastases from primary anal cancers respond no differently to combinations of radiation, 5-FU, and mitomycin and that patients with such metastases can be included in these treatment programs.

Mitomycin was generally given as a bolus injection of 10–15 mg/m^2 either once or twice during the treatment course in these multiple-agent protocols (table 7). This dose is somewhat less than the 20 mg/m^2 recommended as a starting dose for patients receiving mitomycin via an intermittent bolus schedule [12]. The doses of mitomycin given in the treatment schedules shown in table 7 were established empirically and have not been subject to formal studies designed to determine the drug's toxicity when combined with 5-FU and radiation.

The mechanisms of any interactions between radiation and cytotoxic drugs such as mitomycin and 5-FU are unclear, particularly in clinical practice. It is not known whether there is synergism or whether the various agents are simply additive, both in their effects on anal cancer and on normal tissue. The complexities of possible interactions between radiation and cytotoxic drugs have been reviewed by Fu [13] and by Steel [14]. Laboratory evidence both favors [15] and negates [16] synergism between radiation and mitomycin. Mitomycin has demostrated relatively greater toxicity against hypoxic than against normally oxygenated tumor cells [17], although no information exists on the proportion of hypoxic cells present in epidermoid anal cancers, or on whether this characteristic can be exploited in clinical practice. Dobrowsky and Rauth [personal commun., April 1990] indicated that a possible synergism between 5-FU and mitomycin, but not between each of these agents and radiation, in an in vitro mammalian cell system offers an alternative explanation for the apparent importance of mitomycin in our clinical studies.

Some clinical data suggest that different results may be obtained if mitomycin and 5-FU are given sequentially to radiation rather than concurrently. Michaelson et al. [18] and Secco et al. [19] reported series in which a 5-day infusion of 5-FU (750 mg/m^2/24 h) was combined either with a single bolus injection of mitomycin (15 mg/m^2) [18] or with a 12-hour infusion of mitomycin (15 mg/m^2) [19] over 5 days just prior to pelvic irradiation (30 Gy in 15 fractions over 3 weeks). In these series the primary tumor regressed completely in 53% (16 of 30) and 21% (3 of 14) of patients, respectively; both rates were less than the 85% complete regression obtained when similar doses of radiation and chemotherapy were given concurrently [20, 21]. Although there are also other differences between the various series, these results have tended to support the preference for administering 5-FU and mitomycin concurrently with radiation.

There is no evidence in our series that 2 doses of mitomycin at 10 mg/m^2 had any influence as systemic adjuvant therapy. Extrapelvic metastases were found in 17% (8 of 47) of patients who had received two courses of mitomycin and 5-FU, and in 10% (6 of 62) treated with two infusions of 5-FU only. These rates are similar to those reported for patients receiving radiation alone [4], low-dose radiation, 5-FU, and mitomycin [20] and abdominoperineal resection [22]. Michaelson et al. [18] gave multiple courses of 5-FU and mitomycin as adjuvant therapy for up to 1 year to patients who had residual cancer at surgery after preoperative treatment with both agents plus radiation. Recurrence rates were similar whether or not patients received the postoperative adjuvant chemotherapy, and those treated postoperatively experienced significant morbidity, including myelosuppression, azotemia, and microangiopathic hemolytic anemia. These findings were disappointing, as the same authors also reported a 59% response rate (complete plus partial) to 5-FU and mitomycin in patients with advanced anal cancer [18].

Our studies in sequential groups of patients suggest that mitomycin significantly improves eradication of epidermoid anal canal cancers when added to the schedules of radiation and 5-FU used. It will be of interest to see if this observation is confirmed by the as yet uncompleted RTOG randomized trial.

References

1 Nigro ND, Vaitkevicius VK, Herskovic AM: Preservation of function in the treatment of cancer of the anus; in DeVita VT, Hellman S, Rosenberg SA (eds): Important Advances in Oncology. Philadelphia, Lippincott, 1989, pp 161–177.

2 Morson BC, Sobin JH: Histologic typing of intestinal tumors; in International Histological Classification of Tumors. Geneva, World Health Organization, 1976, No 15, pp 62–63.

3 Union Internationale Contre le Cancer: Anal Canal; in Hermanek P, Sobin LH (eds): TNM Classification of Malignant Tumors, ed 4. Berlin, Springer-Verlag, 1987, pp 50–52.

4 Cummings BJ, Keane TJ, O'Sullivan B, et al: Epidermoid anal cancer: Treatment by radiation alone or by radiation and 5-fluorouracil with and without mitomycin C. Int J Radiat Oncol Biol Phys 1991;21:1115–1125.

5 Cummings BJ, Keane TJ, Thomas GM, et al: Results and toxicity of the treatment of anal canal carcinoma by radiation therapy or radiation therapy and chemotherapy. Cancer 1984;54:2062–2068.

6 Ciampi A, Hogg S, McKinney S, et al: RECPAM: A computer program for recursive partition and amalgamation for censored survival data and other situations frequently occurring in biostatistics. Comput Methods Programs Biomed 1988;26:239–256.

7 Flam MS, John MJ, Mowry PA, et al: Definitive combined modality therapy of carcinoma of the anus. Dis Colon Rectum 1987;30:495–502.

8 Sischy B, Lefkopoulou M, Mittelman A, et al: Interim report of EST 7283: A phase II study to evaluate the effectiveness of 5-FU and mitomycin C combined with irradiation in the management of carcinoma of the anal canal (abstract). Proc Am Soc Clin Oncol 1988;7:107.
9 Papillon J, Montbarbon JF: Epidermoid carcinoma of the anal canal. A series of 276 cases. Dis Colon Rectum 1987;30:324–333.
10 Nigro ND, Vaitkevicius VK, Considine B: Combined therapy for cancer of the anal canal. Dis Colon Rectum 1974;17:354–356.
11 Sischy B, Doggett RLS, Krall JM, et al: Definitive irradiation and chemotherapy for radiosensitization in management of anal carcinoma: Interim report on Radiation Therapy Oncology Group Study No. 8314. JNCI 1989;81: 850–856.
12 Crooke ST, Bradner WT: Mitomycin C: A review. Cancer Treat Rev 1976;3:121–139.
13 Fu KK: Biological basis for the interaction of chemotherapeutic agents and radiation therapy. Cancer 1985;55:2123–2130.
14 Steel GG: The search for therapeutic gain in combination of radiotherapy and chemotherapy. Radiother Oncol 1988;11:31–53.
15 Siemann DW, Keng PC: Responses of tumor cell subpopulations to single modality and combined modality therapies. NCI Monogr 1988;6:101–105.
16 Rockwell S: Cytotoxicities of mitomycin-C and x-rays to aerobic and hypoxic cells in vitro. Int J Radiat Oncol Biol Phys 1982;8:1035–1039.
17 Sartorelli AC: Therapeutic attack of hypoxic cells of solid tumors. Cancer Res 1988;48:775–778.
18 Michaelson RA, Magill CB, Quan SHQ, et al: Preoperative chemotherapy and radiation therapy in the management of anal epidermoid carcinoma. Cancer 1983;51:390–395.
19 Secco GB, Sertoli MR, Scarpati D, et al: Preoperative chemotherapy and radiotherapy in the management of epidermoid carcinoma of the anal canal. Tumori 1987;73:151–153.
20 Nigro ND: An evaluation of combined therapy for squamous cell cancer of the anal canal. Dis Colon Rectum 1984;27:763–766.
21 Meeker WR, Sickle-Santanello BJ, Philpott G, et al: Combined chemotherapy, radiation and surgery for epithelial cancer of the anal canal. Cancer 1986;57:525–529.
22 Boman BM, Moertel CG, O'Connell MJ, et al: Carcinoma of the anal canal. A clinical and pathological study of 188 cases. Cancer 1984; 54:114–125.

Oncology 1993;50(suppl 1):70–77

Sandra Schnall
John S. Macdonald

Temple University Comprehensive Cancer Center, Philadelphia, Pa., USA

Mitomycin Therapy in Gastric Cancer

Key Words
Gastric cancer
Mitomycin

Abstract
Adenocarcinoma of the stomach remains a significant cause of mortality worldwide. The majority of patients present with stage III or IV disease, negating surgery as a curative option. Numerous drugs have been tested over the past 2 decades in single-agent and combination chemotherapy trials. Given by intravenous bolus, mitomycin has induced responses as high as 63% and as low as 24% in patients with various gastrointestinal malignancies. Mitomycin has also demonstrated efficacy when given in combination with doxorubicin and in the three-drug regimen FAM (5-fluorouracil/doxorubicin/mitomycin). FAM has been explored in multiple phase II and III trials and has become the standard with which many new combinations are compared. Compared with other doxorubicin-containing regimens, it has demonstrated the longest median survival (29.5 weeks) and the lowest incidence of severe toxicity. The addition of semustine or leucovorin to FAM has yielded responses comparable with those attained by FAM alone. In Japan, where treatment of gastric cancer has been more successful, possibly due to earlier diagnosis and more aggressive surgical approaches, mitomycin has been given intraperitoneally during surgery and postoperatively in combination with fluorinated pyrimidines or other agents. Mitomycin will undoubtedly play a role in the development of new approaches to the treatment of gastric cancer.

Adenocarcinoma of the stomach remains a significant cause of mortality worldwide despite a decline in incidence in the United States and other Western countries. In the United States, gastric cancer is the seventh most common cause of cancer death, whereas in Japan it represents the single greatest cause of cancer mortality [1].

Surgery is the only potentially curative therapy for patients with gastric cancer, and is only effective in localized stomach cancer. Unfortunately, as many as 60% of patients in Western countries present with locally advanced (stage III) or advanced (stage IV) disease at diagnosis, negating surgical therapy as a curative option. Most of these patients die of cancer within 1 year of diagnosis [2]. Therefore, most patients with advanced stomach cancer could benefit from effective chemotherapy.

During the last 20 years numerous chemotherapeutic agents have been evaluated as single agents and in combination in patients with gastric carcinoma [3]. Although single-agent response rates have varied from 1 to 36%, they rarely result in a complete response (CR). One of the more widely used agents both alone and in combination is mitomycin. We will review the role of mitomycin in gastric carcinoma.

Sandra Schnall, MD
Temple University Comprehensive Cancer Center
3322 N. Broad Street
Philadelphia, PA 19140 (USA)

0030–2414/93/0507–0070
$2.75/0

Table 1. Mitomycin in two-drug regimens in patients with gastric cancer

Authors	Ref.	Drug combination	Number of responders/ number of patients	Response, %	Median duration of survival months
Dalley et al.	9	Doxorubicin/mitomycin	4/30	13	3.5
Douglass et al.	10	Doxorubicin/mitomycin	13/46	29	3.5
Buroker et al.	8	5-FU/mitomycin	6/43	14	6.0
Moertel and Lavin	12	5-FU/mitomycin	17/53	32	4.0
O'Connell et al.	11	Triazinate/mitomycin	9/33	27	5.1

Single-Agent Mitomycin

Mitomycin, an antibiotic with a broad spectrum of antitumor activity [4], has been employed mainly in gastrointestinal malignancies. As a single agent given by bolus, mitomycin has induced overall response rates as high as 63% [5] in patients with various gastrointestinal tumors. Other studies, however, have shown less promising results with only a 24% overall response rate [6]. In Japan, mitomycin given on a daily bolus schedule or via continuous infusion yielded promising response rates. Severe cumulative bone marrow toxicity, however, was prohibitive [6, 7].

Mitomycin in Combination Chemotherapy

The evolution of chemotherapeutic treatment of most malignancies has led to the use of combination therapy. In employing several active agents, such an approach may result in increased response rates, duration of response, and overall survival.

Mitomycin has been used in several two-drug combinations (table 1) [8–12]. In 1979 the Southwest Oncology Group (SWOG) conducted a randomized trial that compared a 96-hour infusion of 5-fluorouracil (5-FU) in combination with either bolus mitomycin or orally administered semustine [8]. Ninety-eight patients were enrolled. Of the 97 evaluable patients, 6 of 43 (14%) responded in the mitomycin arm and 5 of 54 (9%) responded in the semustine arm. Median survival for the mitomycin and semustine groups was 25 and 18 weeks, respectively. There was no significant survival difference.

The single-agent response rates of 20–25% [3] obtained with doxorubicin made it a logical choice for evaluation in combination chemotherapy in stomach cancer. Dalley et al. [9] studied doxorubicin in combination with mitomycin in 30 previously untreated patients with advanced gastric cancer. In this phase II trial, patients received doxorubicin 50 mg/m^2 every 3 weeks and mitomycin 10 mg/m^2 every 6 weeks. The overall objective response rate was only 13% with a median survival of 14 weeks. Myelosuppression was the most significant toxicity. When the Eastern Cooperative Oncology Group (ECOG) evaluated this combination in a randomized four-arm trial in advanced gastric cancer, however, response rates of 29 and 21% were noted in previously untreated and previously treated patients, respectively [10]. In this trial doxorubicin was administered at 35 mg/m^2 every 3 weeks and mitomycin at 12 mg/m^2 every 6 weeks. Perhaps the 20% escalated dose of mitomycin yielded a better dose-response effect accounting for the improved response rates.

Baker's antifol, triazinate, has been shown to produce objective tumor responses in 15% of patients with advanced gastric cancer [3]. Investigators at the Mayo Clinic gave combined triazinate and mitomycin to 33 patients, 29 of whom were previously treated, and noted an objective tumor response in 31% [11]. Since previously treated patients are relatively refractory to chemotherapy, the 31% response rate suggested that this regimen should be tested in previously untreated patients.

5-FU/Doxorubicin/Mitomycin Combination Chemotherapy

Perhaps the most widely used regimen with which many new combinations have compared is FAM (5-FU/doxorubicin/mitomycin), which was developed by investigators at the Georgetown Lombardi Cancer Research Center in 1979 [13]. In the initial study of this regimen (table 2), 26 of 62 patients (42%) achieved a partial response (PR) [14]. Median duration of response was 9 months. Median survival was 17.5 months for responders versus 6.5 months for nonresponders. No significant difference was noted between responding and nonresponding patients with reference to performance status, extent of tumor, or site of disease, thereby eliminating the possibility of any bias toward good prognostic features in responding patients.

Table 2. FAM regimen: Schedule of administration (initial phase II trial)

Drug	Dose mg/m²	Route	Week of therapy 1	2	3	4	5	6	7	8	9
5-FU	600	i.v.	×	×			×	×			×
Doxorubicin	30	i.v.	×				×				×
Mitomycin	10	i.v.	×								×

i.v. = Intravenously.

Table 3. FAM regimens in gastric cancer

Authors	Ref.	Number of responders/ number of patients	Response, %	Median duration of survival months
Bitran et al.	20	6/11	55	16.5
Macdonald et al.	14	26/62	42	12.5
Beretta et al.	16	20/45	44	11.5
SWOG	17	6/27	22	5.5
Cunningham et al.	18	28/81	35	17.0
Haim et al.	19	7/33	21	5.5
Haim et al.	15	4/22	18	6.2
Panettiere et al.	21	25/83	30	5.8
GITSG	22	3/12	25	6.8
GITSG	23	3/18	17	6.2
Douglass et al.	10	18/46	39	6.4
Cullinan et al.	24	5/13	38	7.2
Total		151/453	33	

Table 4. Intensified FAM schedule

Drug	Dose mg/m²	Route	Week of therapy 1	2	3	4	5	6	7	8	9
5-FU	600	i.v.	×	×		×	×		×		
Doxorubicin	30	i.v.	×			×			×		
Mitomycin	10	i.v.	×						×		

i.v. = Intravenously.

Since the above results were published, FAM has been explored in multiple phase II and III trials (table 3) [10, 14–24]. Response rates vary from 17 to 55%, with an average PR rate of 33%; CRs, however, have been rare (2% average). It is important to note that several of these trials used doses and schedules other than those described in the initial phase II trial of FAM. The Gastrointestinal Tumor Study Group (GITSG), for example, modified the dose and schedule of 5-FU administration (FAMi), decreasing the dose to 275 mg/m² given daily on days 1–5; doxorubicin was given at 30 mg/m² every 5 weeks and mitomycin at 10 mg/m² every 10 weeks [22, 23]. This schedule resulted in a maximum 25% response rate.

Other modifications of the FAM regimen have been designed to increase dose intensity. Haim et al. [15] shortened the cycle from 8 to 6 weeks (table 4), and noted an overall response rate of 18% in patients with advanced gastric cancer. In most patients this schedule was relatively well tolerated, with a minimal need for increasing intervals between treatments and/or reducing doses. The results, however, suggest that dose intensification did not produce a better response than the original FAM schedule.

SWOG [21] performed a study to determine whether kinetically designed sequential administration of FAM would be superior to traditional FAM. Patients were randomized to receive traditional FAM (table 2) [14] or a sequential schedule in which doxorubicin was given at 50 mg/m² on day 1, mitomycin at 10 mg/m² on day 3, and 5-FU at 600 mg/m² on days 29, 30, 31, and 32. Results showed no statistical difference in overall response rate, 30 versus 23%, between traditional and sequential FAM, respectively.

Several randomized trials have also been completed, which compared the FAM regimen with other combinations in patients with advanced gastric cancer (table 5) [10, 22–24]. The GITSG reported the results of a multicenter clinical trial comparing FAMi, FAMe (5-FU/doxorubicin/semustine), FIMe (5-FU/CRI-159/semustine), and FMe (5-FU/semustine) [22]. One hundred eighty-one patients were evaluated, of whom 59 had measurable indicator lesions. Objective responses were noted in 25, 30, 21, and 6% of patients with measurable disease in the FAMi, FAMe, FIMe, and FMe arms, respectively; median survival rates for these patients were 29.6, 34.4, 17.4, and 22.9 weeks. Toxicity primarily consisted of gastrointestinal side effects and myelosuppression. Patients in both the FAMi and FAMe arms showed improved survival.

Based on the above results, which indicated a possible advantage for the doxorubicin-containing arms, the GITSG proposed a randomized trial comparing FAMi, FAMe, and FA (5-FU/doxorubicin) [23]. Response rates for FAMi and FAMe were 17 and 25%, respectively; overall median survival was 25.7 versus 28.4 weeks. Toxicity was primarily hematologic and seen more commonly in patients receiving FAMe. There was felt to be a slight

Table 5. Randomized trials using FAM

Authors	Ref.	Regimen	Number of responders/number of patients	Response, %	Median duration of survival, weeks
Douglass et al.	10	FMe vs.	6/44	14	13.5
		FAMe vs.	11/39	29	24.5
		FAM vs.	18/46	39	29.5
		AM	13/46	29	19.0
GITSG	22	FAMi vs.	3/12[1]	25	29.6
		FAMe vs.	3/10[1]	30	34.4
		FIMe vs.	4/19[1]	21	17.4
		FMe	1/18[1]	6	22.9
GITSG	23	FA	NR/78	5[1]	25.2
		FAMe vs.	NR/76	25[1]	28.4
		FAMi	NR/78	17[1]	25.7
Cullinan et al.	24	5-FU vs.	2/11[1]	18	29.0
		FA vs.	3/11[1]	27	30.0
		FAM	5/13[1]	38	30.0

NR = Not recorded.
[1] Measurable disease patients only.

survival advantage to the FAMe regimen. It should be noted, however, that the FAMi used by the GITSG and the FAM regimen employ different schedules of 5-FU, which possibly accounted for the difference in response rates.

ECOG compared four different drug regimens in advanced gastric cancer: FMe, FAMe, FAM, and AM (doxorubicin/mitomycin) [10]. Response rates were 14, 29, 39, and 29%, respectively. Patients given FAM had the longest median survival (29.5 weeks) and the lowest incidence of severe toxicity. The results obtained by ECOG are not comparable with those reported by the GITSG since different treatment schedules were employed. Perhaps the lower response rates and increased toxicity in the GITSG study reflect these adjustments.

Three-Drug Combination Chemotherapy

The Georgetown Lombardi Cancer Center designed a trial substituting tegafur for 5-FU in a regimen designated FAM II [25, 26]. Tegafur is an analogue in which 5-FU is conjugated to a furanyl ring. Pharmacologically, the drug acts as a slow-release form of 5-FU, and may cause less marrow toxicity than bolus 5-FU. The regimen consisted of an 8-week cycle, with doxorubicin given at 40 mg/m^2 intravenously on days 1 and 29, mitomycin at 10 mg/m^2 i.v. on day 1, and tegafur at 1.5–2.0 mg/m^2 i.v. on days 1–5 and 29–33. The study demonstrated a 20% response rate among the 15 patients studied. There was increased CNS toxicity and more severe nausea and vomiting with FAM II than with traditional FAM. FAM II was therefore not considered for further investigation.

Epidoxorubicin, a new doxorubicin analogue with relatively less cardiotoxicity than doxorubicin, has been substituted for that drug in FAM, producing a regimen designated FEM. Results of a phase II trial with FEM in patients with advanced gastric cancer were reported in 1986 [27]. A 30% PR rate was achieved among 38 patients studied; there were no CRs. Median survival was 9.3 months for responders and 4.7 months for nonresponders. Although FEM did not show improved activity over FAM, the authors noted that dose escalation of epidoxorubicin was possible. Other studies also using FEM in advanced gastric cancer have shown similar results [28, 29].

Cocconi et al [30] performed an interesting study combining mitomycin, 5-FU, and cytarabine to create a regimen designated MFC. Patients were randomized to receive either 5-FU weekly or MFC. Patients receiving 5-FU alone suffered more severe gastrointestinal toxicity, whereas patients receiving MFC had greater bone marrow suppression. Overall response rates were similar in both arms, 21% for 5-FU versus 28% for MFC.

The GITSG compared MFC with doxorubicin alone or FAMe in patients with advanced gastric cancer [31]. The response rate to MFC was only 9%. The dose schedule employed, however, varied from that used by Cocconi et al. [30], which may explain the difference in therapeutic activity. A phase III study of FAM versus MFC has not been undertaken.

Table 6. Four-drug combinations

Authors	Ref.	Regimen	Number of responders/ number of patients	Response, %	Median duration of survival, months
Karlin et al.	32	FAM/semustine	12/35	34	7.1
Gisselbrecht et al.	33	FAM/chlorozotocin	6/23	26	2.5
Delisi et al.	34	FAM/carmustine	9/41	22	6.0
Beretta et al.	35	FAM/carmustine	5/16	32	NA
Kim and Kim	36	Mitomycin/carmustine/ cisplatin/5-FU	25/38	66	NA
Ahlgren et al.	37	FAM/triazinate	4/34	13	9.0
Arbuck et al.	38	FAM/leucovorin	10/26	38	6.8
Zaniboni et al.	39	FAM/leucovorin	9/19	47	NA

NA = Not available.

Four-Drug Regimens

In an effort to improve survival and response rates of patients with advanced gastric cancer, the FAM regimen has been expanded with the addition of other active chemotherapeutic agents in phase I and II trials (table 6) [32–39].

Karlin et al. [32] evaluated the addition of semustine to FAM (FAMMe) in patients with advanced adenocarcinoma of the upper gastrointestinal tract. Of 115 patients entered, 35 were evaluable for response. Twelve patients (34%) achieved a response, one of whom had a CR. Myelosuppression was the sole dose-limiting toxic effect. Randomized trials comparing FAMMe with other established regimens will be required to confirm the efficacy noted in this trial.

The Georgetown Lombardi Cancer Center, in conjunction with the Hospital St. Louis in Paris, conducted a phase II trial incorporating chlorozotocin in the FAM regimen [33]. Chlorozotocin, a chloroethyl nitrosourea conjugated to a sugar ring structure, has been associated with less myelosuppression than have other chloroethyl nitrosoureas. In this trial, 6 of 23 patients (26%) receiving FAM/chlorozotocin achieved a PR, but there were no CRs. Responses were brief, ranging from 2 to 5 months. These results were inferior to those obtained with FAM alone, even though the absolute doses of FAM given in both regimens were similar. However, dose sequencing may have played a role in this trial's outcome. Other nitrosoureas have been added to the FAM regimen with no combination emerging as superior to FAM [34, 35]. It is doubtful that nitrosoureas will be widely explored, however, due to their leukemogenic potential.

A very promising study reported in abstract form combined 5-FU, carmustine, mitomycin, and cisplatin [36]. Among 38 patients, 25 (66%) had a PR. Survival duration has not been determined. Obviously, the efficacy of this regimen needs to be confirmed in larger trials.

The combination of triazinate with mitomycin has demonstrated activity in advanced gastric cancer [11]. In hopes of exploiting the modulation of 5-FU by antifols, triazinate was added to the original FAM regimen and given 1 h before 5-FU on days 1 and 29 [37]. Investigators noted 3 PRs and 1 CR among 31 evaluable patients, for an overall response rate of 13%. The results were disappointing and inferior to those obtained with FAM alone.

Leucovorin has been shown to enhance the activity of 5-FU through tighter binding of the fluorodeoxyuridine monophosphate (FdUMP)-reduced folate complex to thymidylate synthase (TS), leading to the prolonged inhibition of TS essential to DNA synthesis. Arbuck et al. [38] at Roswell Park Institute evaluated 28 patients with advanced gastric carcinoma with FAM plus leucovorin in a nonrandomized trial. The response rate was 38% with a median survival of 6.8–11.5 months. The dose-limiting toxicity was myelosuppression, necessitating a gradual decrease in 5-FU doses. These results are comparable to those seen with standard FAM.

A similar study from Italy using FAM/leucovorin yielded a response rate of 47% [39]. The authors did not state whether the dose had to be modified due to myelosuppression. Further randomized trials with FAM/leucovorin are warranted.

Combined Modality Therapy

Radiation therapy has curative potential in patients with residual gastric carcinoma. Since chemotherapy is capable of causing regression of advanced gastric cancer, combining radiation with chemotherapy appears an appropriate strategy. Several trials have used mitomycin-based regimens with external beam radiation therapy. The Georgetown Lombardi Cancer Center reported a phase II trial of combined modality therapy using FAM before and after a split course of radiation therapy [40]. Median survival for patients with advanced gastric cancer was 13 months. The treatment was well tolerated. Other trials [41, 42] using FAM and radiation have reported similar median survival rates, despite varying the sequence of the two modalities.

Adjuvant Therapy

Due to the generally high likelihood of relapse after 'curative' surgery in patients with gastric cancer – most notably when the tumor invades the serosa and/or lymph nodes – the use of adjuvant chemotherapy remains an appealing option, especially since chemotherapy has produced good overall responses in advanced disease. Several multicenter trials of adjuvant chemotherapy in gastric cancer have been reported in the United States over the last 15 years. Early studies by the Veterans Administration Surgical Oncology Group (VASOG) [43] and ECOG [44] employing 5-FU and semustine showed no survival advantage. The GITSG [45], however, demonstrated an inprovement in survival in patients given the same agents.

The role of FAM in the adjuvant setting has also been explored. Definitive results of a SWOG phase III study [46] of 221 cases using FAM for six cycles postoperatively in cases with completely resected gastric cancer showed no survival advantage. The British Stomach Cancer Group [47] also reported negative results in a three-arm randomized trial. The International Collaborative Cancer Group [48] recently reported a phase III study using FAM as adjuvant therapy. Three-hundred fifteen patients with gastric cancer were randomized to receive either postoperative treatment with FAM for six cycles or no adjuvant therapy. The interim evaluation suggested evidence of a survival advantage for patients with stage T_3 or T_4 lesions receiving FAM [49–51]. Overall, 56% of patients in the treatment arm and 61% in the observation arm have died. Based on log-rank testing, long-term follow-up demonstrated a continual survival advantage for treated patients with T_3 or T_4 tumors. The authors, however, recommended that these results be viewed with caution, as the data were derived from a retrospective analysis rather than prospective stratification.

A Spanish trial randomized patients postoperatively to treatment with mitomycin 20 mg/m^2 for four courses or observation alone [52]. Among the 70 evaluable patients, fewer relapses occurred in the treatment arm, which also showed improved 5-year survival. Again, these findings were most significant in patients with stage T_3 tumors.

As mentioned earlier, gastric carcinoma is almost endemic in Japan. Fortunately, a larger proportion of Japanese patients are long-term survivors. This has been felt to be secondary to early diagnosis and aggressive surgical approaches. Also, gastric cancer in Japan is often diagnosed at an earlier stage (I or II) than in the United States [53]. Tumors are often less anaplastic and may be associated with intestinal metaplasia. A proportion of improved survival may also be a result of intense adjuvant therapy. Douglass [53] summarized the Japanese approach. Most trials include mitomycin in combination with fluorinated pyrimidines [54]. Patients are often given an intraperitoneal dose of mitomycin at surgery, followed by immediate postoperative chemotherapy.

The Japanese have also explored the use of chemoimmunotherapy in postoperative gastric cancer patients. Ochiai et al. [55] reported results of a randomized controlled study using combination 5-FU, mitomycin, and cytarabine with or without bacille Calmette Guérin/cell wall skeleton. Improved 1-year survival was noted in 65.3% of patients with residual tumor at gastrectomy in the chemoimmunotherapy arm versus 26% of patients treated with chemotherapy alone.

Another Japanese study [56], in which mitomycin plus tegafur, a fluorinated pyrimidine, was compared with mitomycin/tegafur/levamisole, supported Ochiai's results. The tegafur study showed that patients with residual disease postgastrectomy have an improved 2-year survival with chemoimmunotherapy (90%) versus chemotherapy alone (50%). The study should be viewed with caution, however, as one third of patients were excluded from evaluation.

Regional Chemotherapy

Local regional chemotherapy alone has yet to be proven superior to more conventional modalities. Theoretically, this approach allows achievemet of higher localized drug concentrations with less systemic toxicity. The pharmacokinetics of intraperitoneal mitomycin have been studied in clinical trials, which have determined that the maximally tolerated intraperitoneal dose is only 10 mg [57, 58]. The Japanese have been quite innovative in their use of intraperitoneal mitomycin at the time of surgery [53]. They continue to follow this approach in many gastric cancer trials.

A novel approach to intracavitary therapy was described by Hagiwara et al. [59] using mitomycin bound to activated carbon particles (MMC-CH). This approach was designed secondary to evidence that mitomycin injected directly into the peritoneal cavity is easily absorbed, making it difficult to maintain a high drug concentration there [57]. Patients with ascites secondary to various tumors were treated, including 15 with gastric cancer. The use of MMC-CH allowed for slower systemic absorption of mitomycin. An overall response, defined as a decrease in fluid accumulation and improved subjective symptoms, was recorded in 58% of patients with gastric cancer and 82% of patients with pleural effusions.

Another innovative method for controlling local regional recurrence of gastric cancer employed continuous hyperthermic peritoneal perfusion of a solution containing mitomycin (CHPP-M) [60]. Patients had macroscopic serosal invasion but no macroscopic peritoneal metastases after curative surgery for gastric cancer. In this randomized trial 83% of patients treated with CHPP-M were alive at 30 months versus 67.3% of the control group. Although survival was not statistically improved, peritoneal recurrence decreased.

Mitomycin has also been encapsulated in albumin or starch microspheres and successfully infused intra-arterially in Japan [61]. A recent report from Europe [62] confirmed these positive results in the treatment of patients with hepatic metastases from colon cancer. Therapeutic studies have not been reported.

Conclusion

Overall, the role of mitomycin in patients with advanced gastric carcinoma has evolved from its use as a single agent to its current deployment in combination therapy, adjuvant therapy, and novel regional approaches. As newer avenues of treatment, including innovative chemotherapy and combined modality approaches, are developed, it is likely that mitomycin will continue to be a useful agent in gastric cancer chemotherapy.

References

1 Boring CC, Squires TS, Tong T: Cancer Statistics 1991;41:19–39.
2 Macdonald JS, Steele G Jr, Gunderson LL: Cancer of the stomach; in DeVita VT Jr, Hellman S, Rosenberg SA (eds): Cancer Principles and Practices of Oncology, ed 3. Philadelphia, Lippincott, 1989, pp 765–799.
3 Macdonald JS, Gohmann JJ: Chemotherapy of advanced gastric cancer: Present status, future prospects. Semin Oncol 1988;15:42–49.
4 Chabner BA, Myers CE: Clinical pharmacology of cancer chemotherapy; in DeVita VT Jr, Hellman S, Rosenberg SA (eds): Cancer Principles and Practices of Oncology, ed 3. Philadelphia, Lippincott, 1989, pp 349–395.
5 Comis S: Integration of chemotherapy into combined modality treatment of solid tumors. Cancer Treat Rep 1974;1:221–238.
6 Schein PS, Macdonald JS, Hoth D, et al: Mitomycin-C: Experience in the United States with emphasis on gastric cancer. Cancer Chemother Pharmacol 1978;1:73–75.
7 Yap HY, Valdivieso M, Blumenschein G, et al: A phase I-II study of continuous 5-day infusion mitomycin-C. Am J Clin Oncol 1983;6: 109–112.
8 Buroker T, Kim PN, Groppe C, et al: 5-FU infusion with mitomycin-C vs. 5-FU infusion with methyl-CCNU in the treatment of advanced upper gastrointestinal cancer. Cancer 1979;44:1215–1221.
9 Dalley D, Erlichman C, Fine S: Treatment of advanced gastric carcinoma with mitomycin and doxorubicin. Cancer Treat Rep 1986;70: 897–898.
10 Douglass HO Jr, Lavin PT, Goudsmit A, et al: An Eastern Cooperative Oncology Group evaluation of combinations of methyl-CCNU, mitomycin-C, Adriamycin, and 5-fluorouracil in advanced measurable gastric cancer (EST 2277). J Clin Oncol 1984;2:1372–1381.
11 O'Connell MJ, Schutt AJ, Moertel CG, et al: Phase II clinical trial of triazinate in combination with mitomycin-C for patients with advanced gastric cancer. J Clin Oncol 1987;5:83–85.
12 Moertel CG, Lavin PT: Phase II chemotherapy studies in advanced gastric cancer. Cancer Treat Rep 1979;63:1863–1869.
13 Macdonald JS, Woolley PV, Smythe T, et al: 5-Fluorouracil, Adriamycin, and mitomycin-C (FAM) combination chemotherapy in the treatment of advanced gastric cancer. Cancer 1979;44:42–47.
14 Macdonald JS, Schein PS, Woolley PV, et al: 5-Fluorouracil, doxorubicin, and mitomycin (FAM) combination chemotherapy for advanced gastric cancer. Ann Intern Med 1980; 93:533–536.
15 Haim N, Epelbaum R, Cohen Y, et al: Further studies on the treatment of advanced gastric cancer by 5-fluorouracil, Adriamycin (doxorubicin), and mitomycin-C (modified FAM). Cancer 1984;54:1999–2002.
16 Beretta G, Fraschini P, Woolley P, et al: The value of FAM polychemotherapy in advanced gastric carcinoma (abstract). Proc Am Soc Clin Oncol 1982;5:103.
17 The Southwest Oncology Group: 5-Fluorouracil, Adriamycin, and mitomycin-C ± vincristine (FAM vs. V-FAM) compared to chlorozotocin, M-AMSA and dihydroxyanthracenedione with unimpressive differences (abstract). Proc Am Soc Clin Oncol 1983;2:122.
18 Cunningham D, Soukop M, McArdle C, et al: Advanced gastric cancer: Experience in Scotland using 5-fluorouracil, Adriamycin and mitomycin-C. Br J Surg 1984;71:673–676.
19 Haim N, Cohen Y, Honigman J, et al: Treatment of advanced gastric carcinoma with 5-fluorouracil, Adriamycin, and mitomycin-C (FAM). Cancer Chemother Pharmacol 1982; 8:277–280.
20 Bitran J, Desser R, Kozloff MK, et al: Treatment of metastatic pancreatic and gastric adenocarcinomas with 5-fluorouracil, Adriamycin, and mitomycin-C (FAM). Cancer Treat Rep 1979;63:2049–2051.

21 Panettiere FJ, Haas C, McDonald B, et al: Drug combinations in the treatment of gastric adenocarcinoma: A randomized Southwest Oncology Group study. J Clin Oncol 1984;2: 420–424.
22 The Gastrointestinal Tumor Study Group: A comparative clinical assessment of combination chemotherapy in the management of advanced gastric carcinoma. Cancer 1982;49: 1362–1366.
23 The Gastrointestinal Tumor Study Group: Randomized study of combination chemotherapy in unresectable gastric cancer. Cancer 1984;53:13–17.
24 Cullinan SA, Moertel CG, Fleming TR, et al: A comparison of three chemotherapeutic regimens in the treatment of advanced pancreatic and gastric carcinoma. JAMA 1985;253:2061–2067.
25 Treat J, Falchuk SC, Woolley PV, et al: Therapy of advanced gastric carcinoma. Am J Clin Oncol 1989;12:162–168.
26 Woolley PV, Macdonald JS, Smythe PA, et al: A phase II trial of Ftorafur. Cancer 1979;44: 1211–1214.
27 Queiber W, Fletchtner H, Henb H, et al: 5-Fluorouracil, 4-epidoxorubicin, and mitomycin-C (FEM) for advanced gastric carcinoma: A phase II trial (abstract). J Cancer Res Clin Oncol 1986;111:85.
28 Roth A, Zupanc D, Lueti CJ, et al: Open phase II trial with 5-fluorouracil, 4-epi-doxorubicin and mitomycin-C (FEM) in advanced gastric cancer. Tumori 1990;79:51–53.
29 Itoh T, Sakata Y, Tamura Y, et al: Effect of combination of 5-fluorouracil, epirubicin, and mitomycin-C (FEM) on advanced gastric carcinoma. J Jpn Soc Cancer Ther 1989;20:1551–1556.
30 Cocconi G, DeLisi V, DiBlasio B: Randomized comparison of 5-FU alone or combined with mitomycin and cytarabine (MFC) in the treatment of advanced gastric cancer. Cancer Treat Rep 1982;66:1263–1266.
31 The Gastrointestinal Tumor Study Group: Phase II–III chemotherapy studies in advanced gastric cancer. Cancer Treat Rep 1979; 63:1871–1876.
32 Karlin DA, Stroehlein JR, Bennetts RW, et al: Phase I-II study of the combination of 5-FU, doxorubicin, mitomycin, and semustine (FAMMe) in the treatment of adenocarcinoma of the stomach, gastroesophageal junction, and pancreas. Cancer Treat Rep 1982;66: 1613–1617.
33 Giesselbrecht C, Smith FP, Macdonald JS, et al: The effect of sequential addition of the nitrosourea, chlorozotocin, to the FAM combination in advanced gastric cancer. Cancer 1983;51:1792–1794.
34 De Lisi V, Cocconi G, Tonato M, et al: Randomized comparison of 5-FU alone or combined with carmustine, doxorubicin, and mitomycin (BAFMi) in the treatment of advanced gastric cancer: A phase III trial of the Italian Clinical Research Oncology Group (GOIRC). Cancer Treat Rep 1986;70:481–485.
35 Beretta G, Fraschini P, Ravaioli A, et al: FAM/FAMB polychemotherapy for advanced carcinoma of the stomach (ACS): A randomized study (abstract). Proc Am Soc Clin Oncol 1983;2:131.
36 Kim RH, Kim CS: Chemotherapy of advanced gastric cancer with mitomycin-C, BCNU, cisplatin, and 5-fluorouracil in combination (abstract). Proc Am Soc Clin Oncol 1986;5:78.
37 Ahlgren JD, Smith FP, Cazap E, et al: FAM (5-fluorouracil, doxorubicin, and mitomycin) plus triazinate (FAM-T) in gastric carcinoma: A combined phase II trial of the Mid-Atlantic Oncology Program and the Pan American Health Organization. Cancer Treat Rep 1987; 71:419–420.
38 Arbuck SG, Silk Y, Douglass HO Jr, et al: A phase II trial of 5-fluorouracil, doxorubicin, mitomycin-C, and leucovorin in advanced gastric carcinoma. Cancer 1990;65:2442–2445.
39 Zaniboni A, Simoncini E, Marpicati P, et al: Mitomycin-C (MMC), Adriamycin (ADM), 5-fluorouracil (5-FU), and folinic acid (FA) in advanced gastric cancer (CG): Preliminary results (abstract). Proc Am Soc Clin Oncol 1989; 8:107.
40 Schein PS, Smith FP, Dritschillo A, et al: Phase I-II trial of combined modality FAM (5-fluorouracil, Adriamycin, and mitomycin-C) plus split course radiation (FAM-RT-FAM) for locally advanced gastric (LAG) and pancreatic (LAP) cancer: A Mid-Atlantic Oncology Program (abstract). Proc Am Soc Clin Oncol 1983;2:126.
41 Audeh WM, Carlson RW, Jacobs CD, et al: Long-term survival in advanced gastric carcinoma following combined modality therapy: The Stanford University experience (abstract). Proc Am Soc Clin Oncol 1989;8:118.
42 Bukowski RM, Theodors A, Purvis JD, et al: Phase II trial of sequential chemotherapy and low-dose radiotherapy in advanced gastric adenocarcinoma. Am J Clin Oncol 1987;10: 376–379.
43 The Veterans Administration Surgical Oncology Group: Efficacy of prolonged intermittent therapy with combined 5-FU and methyl-CCNU following resection for gastric carcinoma. Cancer 1983;52:1105–1112.
44 Engstrom PF, Lavin PT, Douglass HO Jr, et al: Postoperative adjuvant 5-fluorouracil plus methyl-CCNU therapy for gastric cancer patients. Cancer 1985;55:1868–1873.
45 The Gastrointestinal Tumor Study Group: Controlled trial of adjuvant chemotherapy following curative resection for gastric cancer. Cancer 1982;49:1116–1122.
46 Macdonald JS, Gagliano R, Fleming T, et al: A phase III trial of FAM as adjuvant treatment for resected gastric cancer (a Southwest Oncology Group trial – SWOG 7804) (abstract). Proc Am Soc Clin Oncol 1992;11:168.
47 Fielding JWL, Fagg SL, Jones BG, et al: An interim report of a prospective, randomized, controlled study of adjuvant chemotherapy in operable gastric cancer: British Stomach Cancer Group. World J Surg 1983;7:390–399.
48 Coombes RC, Schein PS, Chilvers CED, et al: A randomized trial comparing adjuvant fluorouracil, doxorubicin, and mitomycin with no treatment in operable gastric cancer. J Clin Oncol 1990;8:1362–1369.
49 Rauschecker H, Osterloh B: Is FAM an effective drug regimen in the adjuvant treatment of gastric cancer? (abstract). J Cancer Res Clin Oncol 1986;111:85.
50 Wils J, Coombes RC, Chilvers C, et al: Randomized trial of FAM (5-fluorouracil, Adriamycin, mitomycin-C) chemotherapy versus control as adjuvant treatment for resected gastric cancer: 4, 5 year results (abstract). Proc Am Soc Clin Oncol 1988;7:97.
51 Schein PS, Coombes RC, Chilvers C: A controlled trial of FAM (5-FU, doxorubicin, and mitomycin-C) chemotherapy as adjuvant treatment for resected gastric carcinoma: An interim report (abstract). Proc Am Soc Clin Oncol 1986;5:79.
52 Alcobendas F, Milla A, Estape J, et al: Mitomycin-C as an adjuvant in resected gastric cancer. Ann Surg 1983;198:13–17.
53 Douglass HO Jr: Gastric cancer: Overview of current therapies. Semin Oncol 1985;3:57–62.
54 Inokuchi K, Hattori T, Taguchi T, et al: Postoperative adjuvant chemotherapy for gastric carcinoma, Cancer 1984;53:2393–2397.
55 Ochiai T, Sato H, Hayashi R, et al: Randomly controlled study of chemotherapy versus chemoimmunotherapy in postoperative gastric cancer patients. Cancer Res 1983;43:3001–3007.
56 Niimoto M, Hattori T, Ito T, et al: Levamisole in postoperative adjuvant immunotherapy for gastric cancer. Cancer Immunol Immunother 1984;18:13–18.
57 Gyves J: Pharmacology of intraperitoneal infusion 5-fluorouracil and mitomycin-C. Semin Oncol 1985;3:29–32.
58 Speyer JL: The rationale behind intraperitoneal chemotherapy in gastrointestinal malignancies. Semin Oncol 1985;3:23–28.
59 Hagiwara A, Takahashi T, Lee R, et al: Chemotherapy for carcinomatous peritonitis and pleuritis with MMC-CH, mitomycin-C absorbed on activated carbon particles. Cancer 1987; 59:245–251.
60 Koga S, Hamazoe R, Maeta M, et al: Prophylactic therapy for peritoneal recurrence of gastric cancer by continuous hyperthermic peritoneal perfusion with mitomycin C. Cancer 1988;61:232–237.
61 Fujimoto S, Miyazaki M, Endoh F, et al: Effects of intra-arterially infused biodegradable microspheres containing mitomycin-C. Cancer 1985;55:522–526.
62 Goldberg JA, Kerr DJ, Blackie R, et al: Mitomycin-C loaded microcapsules in the treatment of colorectal liver metastases. Cancer 1991;67:952–955.

Oncology 1993;50(suppl 1):78–83

Clare Topham
J. Glees
R. C. Coombes

St. Luke's Hospital, Guildford, UK

Comparison of Single-Agent Epirubicin and 5-Fluorouracil / Epirubicin / Mitomycin in Patients with Advanced Adenocarcinoma of the Pancreas

Key Words
FEM
Epirubicin
Pancreatic adenocarcinoma

Abstract
In a randomized trial we compared single-agent epirubicin with the FEM (5-fluorouracil/epirubicin/mitomycin) combination in patients with locally advanced and/or metastatic adenocarcinoma of the pancreas. Sixty patients previously untreated with radiotherapy or chemotherapy were randomly assigned to receive either 100 mg/m^2 epirubicin or FEM in the following doses: 5-fluorouracil, 600 mg/m^2 to a maximum of 1 g; epirubicin, 50 mg/m^2; mitomycin, 6 mg/m^2 to a maximum of 10 mg. Treatment was given every 28 days via intravenous bolus; because of its association with delayed myelotoxicity, mitomycin was given every other cycle. A total of 47 patients are evaluable for toxicity and survival, 22 who received FEM and 25 epirubicin. Preliminary results of this ongoing study show no difference in survival between the two arms. Toxicity has been easily managed. A similar number of patients in each arm had elevated serum bilirubin levels, but dose reductions of 50% allowed all these patients to continue treatment.

The 5-year survival of patients with adenocarcinoma of the pancreas has been extremely poor (<2%) [1], primarily because most of these patients present with advanced local disease or distant metastases. The extent of disease has proven difficult to evaluate. Surgery sometimes helps in this measure, and may be used to perform biliary bypass for palliation. Attempts at curative resection are possible in only a small minority of patients. These problems in evaluating the extent of pancreatic cancer have also hindered efforts to devise and assess effective chemotherapeutic strategies. The most thoroughly studied agents to date, 5-fluorouracil (5-FU) and mitomycin have achieved single-agent response rates of 20–30% [1, 2]. Doxorubicin has not fared as well, yielding a 13% response rate [1, 2]. When given in combination in several studies, however, the 3 drugs have produced a consistent overall response of approximately 40%, a median survival for responders of 12 months, and median overall survival of 6 months [2].

In 1985, the European Organization for the Research and Treatment of Cancer reported that epirubicin, a doxorubicin analogue, induced an overall response rate of 24% among patients with advanced pancreatic cancer. Median survival of responders and median overall survival with this analogue were 9 and 5 months, respectively [3]. These findings, coupled with those of a report [4] published the same year that showed epirubicin caused

Clare Topham, MD
St. Luke's Hospital
Warren Road
Guildford, Surrey GU1 3NT (UK)

0030–2414/93/0507–0078
$2.75/0

less acute toxicity – e.g., nausea and vomiting, stomatitis, and myelosuppression – than its parent compound, led us to speculate that epirubicin might also be more effective than doxorubicin when given in combination with 5-FU/mitomycin (FEM) to patients with advanced pancreatic cancer.

A pilot study conducted by Topham [5], in which FEM was given every 28 days to 8 pancreatic cancer patients, showed the regimen to be well tolerated, with no significant hematologic toxicity observed. Side effects consisted of slight alopecia in 3 patients (World Health Organization, WHO, grade 2) and vomiting in 1 (WHO grade 2).

Concluding that FEM could be given safely to pancreatic cancer patients, we commenced a randomized study comparing single-agent epirubicin with FEM in patients with advanced local and/or metastatic disease. Although the study is still accruing patients, we report here our preliminary findings, emphasizing toxicity and survival.

Patients and Methods

Patients had to have histologically confirmed, advanced local and/or metastatic adenocarcinoma of the pancreas previously untreated with chemotherapy or radiotherapy. Other entry criteria are summarized in table 1. Sixty patients were enrolled from the three hospitals within our group. The majority of patients underwent palliative surgery and were stratified into groups of those with and those without liver metastases. Patients were randomly assigned to receive either 100 mg/m^2 epirubicin or FEM in the following doses: 5-FU, 600 mg/m^2 (maximum, 1 g); epirubicin, 50 mg/m^2; mitomycin, 6 mg/m^2 (maximum, 10 mg). Patients with raised serum bilirubin levels were not excluded from treatment, but their drug doses were halved. Treatment was given on an outpatient basis every 28 days via intravenous bolus; because of its association with delayed myelotoxicity, mitomycin was given every other cycle. Blood samples were drawn on day 28, before the next treatment course, to assess hematologic toxicity. Most patients received scalp cooling with chemotherapy. Monthly therapy continued until a patient showed definite signs of disease progression, at which point further treatment was left to the discretion of the investigators. Toxicity was assessed using WHO criteria, survival estimated with life tables, and comparisons between groups were made using the log-rank test. In all, 47 of 60 patients were evaluable for toxicity and survival, 25 of whom received epirubicin and 22 FEM. One patient died before receiving treatment, and data for 3 others were unavailable for analysis; of the remaining 9 patients, 3 patients each were inevaluable due to incorrect histology, previous chemotherapy, and refusal of informed consent. Evaluable patients in both treatment arms were evenly matched for age and sex (table 2). A comparable number of evaluable patients had liver metastases (9 receiving epirubicin, 7 FEM). Time elapsed from diagnosis to treatment is shown in table 3. The median time intervals reflect the study data more closely, since only a few patients went without treatment for long periods after diagnosis. Baseline peripheral blood counts were comparable in each arm. Drug doses had to be reduced by 50% in more than half the patients (similar numbers in each arm) because of elevated serum bilirubin levels (median, 25–30 μmol/l; range, 20–311). The 22 patients in the FEM arm received a total of 94 courses of therapy (median, 2; range, 1–11); 7 patients were given only 1 course. In the epirubicin arm, a total of 83 courses (median, 3; range, 1–10) were given to the 25 patients; 5 patients received only 1 course.

Table 1. Comparison of epirubicin and FEM: Entry criteria

No concomitant psychiatric or uncontrolled cardiovascular disorders
No prior history of malignancy
WBC count $\geq 3.0 \times 10^9$/l
Platelet count $\geq 100 \times 10^9$/l
Serum creatinine <150 μmol/l

WBC = White blood cell.

Table 2. Comparison of epirubicin and FEM: Age and sex of evaluable patients

	FEM (n = 22)	Epirubicin (n = 25)
Mean age, years	62	64
Range	42–78	39–80
Sex, M/F	11/11	15/10

Table 3. Comparison of epirubicin and FEM: Time elapsed from diagnosis

	FEM (n = 22)	Epirubicin (n = 25)
Median time, days	18	27
Range	6–180	6–321

Results

Survival

Twelve patients (26%) died of disease progression within 1 month of study entry, 7 of whom had received FEM and 5 epirubicin. One patient died of myocardial infarction following 10 courses of FEM; the death was not drug-related. There was no significant difference in sur-

Table 4. Comparison of epirubicin and FEM: Nausea and vomiting

	Patients			
	FEM (n = 20)[1]		epirubicin (n = 25)	
WHO Grade	n	%	n	%
None	4	20	11	44
1	6	30	5	20
2	9	45	3	12
3	1	5	6	24

[1] Toxicity grades were not recorded for 2 patients.

vival between the treatment groups. Median survival from start of chemotherapy for patients receiving FEM was 6.6 months versus 5.2 months for patients receiving epirubicin. Overall, median survival for all patients from day of surgery to death was 6.8 months.

Toxicity

White blood cell counts were depressed in 2 patients receiving FEM (WHO grades 1 and 2) compared with 1 (WHO grade 1) receiving epirubicin. Platelet counts remained within normal limits. Grade 1 or 2 hemoglobin toxicity occurred in 2 patients receiving FEM and in 3 receiving epirubicin. An additional patient receiving epirubicin had grade 3 toxicity. The next course of chemotherapy was delayed slightly in these 6 patients for the administration of hemoglobin transfusions (3 or 4 units). The severity of the worst episode of nausea and vomiting is shown in table 4. Often this adverse effect was related to the disease as well as to chemotherapy. Although 80% of patients receiving FEM experienced some degree of nausea and vomiting compared with 56% of those receiving epirubicin, the difference was not statistically significant ($\chi^2 = 1.9$; $0.1 < p < 0.2$). Moreover, there was no discernible difference between treatment arms in the proportion of courses during which toxicity was recorded. Eight of 14 patients receiving epirubicin and 8 of 16 receiving FEM experienced nausea and vomiting with every course. Alopecia occurred in the 5 patients in each arm who had not been treated with cold caps. One patient in each group had nonlife-threatening septicemia; neither episode was related to drug-induced neutropenia.

Conclusion

This small group of patients mirrors the clinical spectrum of adenocarcinoma of the pancreas. The interim results of this ongoing study indicate there is no difference in survival between patients receiving FEM and epirubicin. The toxicity of both regimens is moderate and easily managed. Patients with raised serum bilirubin levels can be treated safely with lower doses of these agents.

References

1 Zimmerman SE, et al: Chemotherapy of pancreatic carcinoma. Cancer 1981;47:1724–1728.

2 Smith FP, et al: 5-Fluorouracil, Adriamycin, and mitomycin-C (FAM) chemotherapy for advanced adenocarcinoma of the pancreas. Cancer 1980;46:2014–2018.

3 Wils J, et al. (for the EORTC Gastrointestinal Group): Phase II study of epirubicin in advanced adenocarcinoma of the pancreas. Eur J Cancer Clin Oncol 1985;21:191–194.

4 Ganzina F, et al: Clinical toxicity of 4′-epi-doxorubicin (epi-rubicin). Tumori 1985;71:233–240.

5 Topham C: Epirubicin in the FEM regimen in cancer of the stomach and pancreas. Clin Trials 1987;24(suppl 1):191–194.

Discussion

Dr. Schnall: Is there still a role for surgery in the treatment of anal canal cancer?

Dr. Keane: There has been a big difference with regard to treatment of anal canal cancer in the United States compared with Europe and certainly Canada. Traditionally, surgery in the form of abdominal perineal resection was widely used in the United States as the treatment of choice for anal canal cancer. This was not so in France, and certainly not in Canada and many places in Britain.

I think it's fair to say that the treatment regimen of concurrent radiotherapy/5-fluorouracil (5-FU)/mitomycin, pioneered by Dr. Nigro, a surgeon at Wayne State University, has completely transformed the treatment of anal canal cancer in the United States. Abdominal perineal resection is now reserved only for patients who are incontinent at presentation, in whom there is no point in attempting to preserve anal rectal function with radiotherapy.

For continent patients, I think radiotherapy/5-FU/mitomycin has become essentially the treatment of choice, although there are many approaches to it. Some physicians, for instance, are using 5-FU/mitomycin/radiotherapy with just a local excision – kind of an extended biopsy – while preserving anal rectal function. But the whole emphasis now has shifted away from abdominal perineal resection, and I think that's widely accepted.

Question: How do you assess local disease control? For example, do you do blind biopsies of the region?

Dr. Keane: No. We have maintained a policy of clinical follow-up and reserve biopsy for those situations in which clinical evidence suggests recurrent disease. Other groups have done random or blind biopsies of the primary tumor site from 2 to 3 months postradiotherapy. We don't see any value in that. We follow these patients very carefully. The anal canal can be examined easily, and disease recurrence can be detected clinically, I think, without difficulty.

Question: Do you attempt to re-treat patients who fail initial treatment with radiation and chemotherapy? Or are they managed surgically at that point?

Dr. Keane: Overall salvage rates following radical-dose radiotherapy have not been impressive. No more than 30–40% of patients who failed the initial regimen had long-term survival following surgical salvage treatment.

Question: Is there any way to improve long-term survival in patients with anal carcinoma? How can we get the projection closer to 100%, which is obviously our goal?

Dr. Keane: The 5-year survival projection for patients with anal canal carcinoma treated with 5-FU/mitomycin/radiotherapy is around 70%. With 90% local disease control, it's going to be very hard to improve that figure. I don't believe you can achieve better than 90% local control at any site with this variety of tumor.

One could argue that patients with stage TI tumors don't need 5-FU/mitomycin – that almost 90% local control can be obtained with radiotherapy alone. The big improvements with the combined-modality regimen are achieved in large tumors. So, given the rarity of this disease, I think it very unlikely – certainly in randomized studies – that one would ever accrue enough patients to have a study with sufficient power to demonstrate actual improvements in local control above the present level.

Dr. Henderson: Dr. Keane, earlier you showed two survival curves comparing results with 5-FU alone and those of 5-FU/mitomycin that showed a rather substantial (suggesting a statistically significant) difference in survival favoring the combination regimen. Was that disease-free survival or cause-specific survival?

Dr. Keane: Cause-specific survival.

Dr. Henderson: Yet there wasn't a significant difference between treated patients and historical controls in terms of extrapelvic recurrence rates, which suggests that the cause of death in these patients with anal carcinoma was local disease. That contradicts what happens in most cancers; most patients die of distant organ disease.

Dr. Keane: Historically, the vast majority of patients with anal canal cancer died of what I call pelvic disease – maybe not confined to the local site but within the pelvis. And I think all the data show that. So when one improves local disease control, one can expect an improvement in survival. I think that's been demonstrated.

I think one has to be careful when attempting to interpret this survival data for several reasons. For one, the control data were compiled over a period of 22 years, and in that time there have been tremendous technologic improvements in our ability to detect and diagnose distant metastases. Also, it could well be that patients with anal carcinoma who die of local disease don't live long enough for distant metastases to occur. Finally, when looking at the number of deaths in a mixed patient population, one has to separate deaths due to anal carcinoma from deaths due to other causes before trying to establish a pattern of failure.

Dr. Sedlacek: With these very good results in anal canal cancer, have you tried using 5-FU/mitomycin/radiotherapy in patients with locally advanced adenocarcinoma of the rectum?

Dr. Keane: We've been involved in studies for the last decade. In addition to the nonrandomized studies in patients with esophageal and anal canal cancer, two major randomized trials of mitomycin/5-FU are under way in patients with squamous cell cancers of the cervix, larynx, and pharynx. So far, the results have not been as impressive. In the case of rectal carcinoma, we did some studies of radiotherapy with 5-FU/mitomycin in the early 1980s and we didn't see anything to suggest this regimen had efficacy comparable with what we later observed in anal canal cancer. Results of pilot studies of 5-FU/mitomycin and simultaneous radiotherapy in advanced bladder and breast cancers have likewise not been as impressive as the results in squamous cell carcinomas of the anal canal.

Dr. Weissberg and his colleagues at Yale did a randomized trial comparing radiotherapy with radiotherapy/mitomycin, using mitomycin as a radiosensitizer, in patients with head and neck squamous carcinoma. Although the trial had a surgical component to it, the addition of mitomycin to the radiotherapy regimen improved local control. The data are very compelling, but it is probably one of the most ignored trials in head and neck cancer because people somehow didn't believe that a single agent given in two doses could have a major effect.

Biologically, mitomycin, because of its unique characteristics as an alkylating agent and a hypoxic cell cytotoxin, has a whole range of potential for radiotherapists that perhaps makes it worth exploring as a single agent.

Dr. Henderson: Doesn't warfarin somehow direct mitomycin in its reductive activation, which leads to greater efficacy of the drug?

Dr. Keane: The drug can be manipulated pharmacologically in a number of interesting ways. Most often mitomycin has been given by a single intravenous bolus injection. Using mitomycin in a different way, certainly combined with concurrent radiotherapy, might open up new areas of research worth developing.

Dr. Henderson: Dr. Schnall, has mitomycin been established, in any of the large studies you summarized, as an agent that, when added to combination chemotherapy, improves overall survival in patients with advanced gastric cancer?

Dr. Schnall: The data show that none of the single-agent or combination chemotherapy regimens used in these trials has significantly improved overall survival in patients with gastric cancer. Relatively high response rates have been obtained, but the survival curves all meet at approximately the same point. So, despite the use of various drug combinations, survival really hasn't been improved.

Dr. Henderson: Do you feel there is convincing evidence at this point that mitomycin improves combination chemotherapy?

Dr. Schnall: A single-agent trial comparing mitomycin with doxorubicin might help clarify which agent shows greater potential as a component of combination chemotherapy. As a single agent in phase I/II trials mitomycin has fared better overall, but it's never been compared in a phase III trial.

Dr. Coia: I was impressed with the 66% overall response rate you said one trial reported for the four-drug combination of cisplatin/mitomycin/carmustine/5-fluorouracil. What toxicities were reported in that trial and how severe were they?

Dr. Schnall: Toxicity was not severe. I think the major toxicity was marrow suppression. But the combination was quite tolerable, and most patients were able to receive two or three cycles without much difficulty.

Dr. Folman: From the perspective of a community oncologist, acknowledging the potential for toxicity with platinum combinations, my question is, what do you recommend for the treatment of gastric cancer? Should you use mitomycin if you're not going to use platinum? From the data presented, my impression is you probably should.

Dr. Schnall: Currently, I recommend using the ELF regimen (etoposide/leucovorin/5-FU) for recurrent gastric carcinoma, which is very easy to administer in an outpatient setting and has been associated with less toxicity in terms of marrow suppression than platinum-based regimens such as EAP (etoposide/doxorubicin/cisplatin). I think ELF might be a very convenient regimen to use, especially in patients with advanced disease. However, based on combination chemotherapy studies, platinum does appear to have respectable response rates in gastric carcinoma. To my knowledge, mitomycin and cisplatin have not been compared as single agents in gastric cancer. To study adjuvant therapy, we have begun a trial in which patients with gastric cancer receive two cycles of 5-FU/leucovorin postoperatively followed by 5-FU/leucovorin with concurrent radiation therapy and then two more cycles of postradiation chemotherapy. I would consider using this regimen in the community setting if the radiation therapist felt comfortable with it.

Dr. Henderson: What is the single-agent activity of etoposide in this disease?

Dr. Schnall: Etoposide has induced overall response rates somewhere between 20 and 30%.

Dr. Hortobagyi: Have any of the gastric cancer studies you mentioned looked at the degree of palliation offered by any of these regimens?

Dr. Schnall: I don't believe so. Some of the more recent Japanese studies assessing new approaches to the use of mitomycin noted improved palliation in terms of ascites and discomfort and some slight improvement in survival, but I don't think any of the larger randomized trials using chemotherapy singled out palliation as a response criterion.

Dr. Sedlacek: Dr. Schnall, please comment on the North Central Onocology Group's study of 5-FU versus 5-FU/doxorubicin versus 5-FU/doxorubicin/mitomycin (FAM) in 300 patients with gastric and pancreatic cancers.

Dr. Schnall: The FAM arm had marginally better response rates but was associated with increased toxicity and cost. There was no improvement in survival in any of the arms.

Dr. Sedlacek: Dr. Robert Dorr and the University of Arizona Cancer Center are looking at the use of megestrol acetate with mitomycin in patients with colon cancer. They have also reported significant reductions in hematologic toxicity when mitomycin is given in doses of, I believe, 3 mg/m^2/day for 5 days by continuous infusion.

Dr. Henderson: In administering that dose by continuous infusion, were both thrombocytopenia and neutropenia decreased?

Dr. Sedlacek: They didn't distinguish between the two. They just said that hematologic toxicity decreased significantly in 6 patients treated so far.

Dr. Keane: Virtually all continuous infusion studies show less hematologic toxicity than is observed with other routes of administration. Do any data demonstrate that continuous infusion mitomycin is of equal efficacy to standard treatment? Or are you just using the drug in a more homeopathic approach?

Dr. Hortobagyi: We did a study in which mitomycin was given at 4 mg/m^2/day by continuous infusion over 5 days to previously treated patients with metastatic breast cancer. The treatment, however, was not effective. Actually, there was no difference in hematologic toxicity whether the drug was given by continuous infusion or in single intermittent high doses. All preclinical data for mitomycin suggest that treatment with single intermittent doses is better than with divided doses. But no comparative trials have been done.

Dr. Schnall: The Southwest Oncology Group is looking at 5-day bolus 5-FU versus continuous infusion 5-FU with modulator variations in patients with advanced colon carcinoma.

Dr. Henderson: I think we can summarize by saying that gastric cancer is one of the areas where mitomycin is most established as an effective drug. Although Dr. Schnall didn't comment on it specifically, we can assume, from the first phase II studies, that mitomycin probably is somewhat non-cross-resistant in patients who've been exposed previously to 5-FU. Mitomycin is probably most widely used in the most established regimen, FAM, but its particular contribution to that regimen is not well defined by currently available data.

Author Index

Subject Index